My Real Life Miracle

My Real Life Miracle

From Nurse to Patient:
My COVID Story and the Miracle that Saved my Life

DR. LISA AMICK
& ELDER DAVID AMICK

XULON PRESS

Xulon Press
2301 Lucien Way #415
Maitland, FL 32751
407.339.4217
www.xulonpress.com

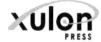

Paperback ISBN-13: 978-1-66287-780-3

Hard Cover ISBN-13: 978-1-66287-781-0
Ebook ISBN-13: 978-1-66287-782-7

Dedication

This book is dedicated to our parents, Billy and Jane (my angel) Russell; Paul (my other angel) and Sheila Amick. You have each supported us and have always had faith in God and loved all your children, grandchildren, and great-grandson unconditionally with all your hearts.

Thank you for setting the example of how to be good Christian followers and setting us on our path to accepting Jesus as our Lord and Savior.

We love you very much.

Introduction

The year 2020 will go down in history as the year of so many unknowns and uncertainties, the year COVID-19 took the world hostage. For the first time in United States history, Americans were ordered to self-isolate: adults were not to go to work, kids were not allowed at school, businesses were forced closed, and chaos erupted. For our family, 2020 went down in history as a year we would rather forget. Things were certainly crazy. The world was imploding! Families were struggling. Slogans like, "We can get through this together," "Together We Will" and "Be safe" had taken over our lives and social media. It was like we were living in the twilight zone, watching some sort of bizarre Quentin Tarantino movie.

We were all wearing masks. Talk about giving the bad guys a break! No one could tell the bad guys from the good guys, giving criminals a free pass. I mean for real, ya'll! Everyone was wearing a mask! It felt like we were all playing Batman and Robin! People thought COVID was some sort of government conspiracy theory to control our minds and our lives. People thought President Trump came up with this to get back at those who were not part of the basket of deplorables. Americans were losing their minds.

It was a nightmare.

Especially for those who were touched on a personal level or in a devastating way.

According to the World Health Organization, there have been 760,897,555 confirmed cases of COVID and 6,874,585 deaths worldwide. In fact, as of early 2023, at the three-year mark, there have been 618,360 new cases confirmed in the last twenty-four hours, and the pandemic is considered over. At least 17 million worldwide suffer from long COVID symptoms—17 million people all over the world just like me.

Scratch your head over those numbers. They are unbelievable.

What is Long COVID, you ask? The US Department of Health and Human Services noted soon after the COVID-19 pandemic began that some patients were not fully recovering. These patients referred to themselves as Long haulers. Even previously healthy patients who contracted COVID were not recovering. This completely threw the healthcare industry for a loop. Why were these patients not fully recovering? There was no rhyme or reason to it. Check out this list of symptoms of Long COVID. Long haulers can have any combination (I will put an asterisk * next to the symptoms I have experienced):

Extreme Fatigue *

Fatigue that gets worse after physical exercise (post-exertional malaise) *

Fever

Shortness of Breath *

Cough *

Chest Pain

Fast beating or pounding heart rate *

Brain Fog (difficulty concentrating) *

Headache *

Sleep problems (insomnia) *

Dizziness *

Pins and Needles sensation *

Change in smell or taste

Depression or Anxiety

Stomach Pain

Joint or Muscle Pain *

Rash

Changes in Menstrual Cycles

Tinnitus *

GI Symptoms *

There are no known treatments for Long COVID, just experimental treatments for symptom management. People who suffer from Long COVID often are made to feel as if they are making everything up. The American Disability Act has recognized Long COVID as a disability, yet a lot of times we are made to feel like we are making all this up. I am often made to feel like this is all in my head. I invite anyone who thinks that to spend one day walking in my shoes. I double-dog dare you.

Let me introduce myself. My name is Dr. Lisa Amick, and I'm a nurse. I have been married for thirty-six years to a wonderful man, David, who also happens to be the co-author of this book. He is a chief technologist in the radiology department at a local Veteran's Hospital where I also work in a leadership position. He is a veteran himself, so working at the VA is personal for both of us. We have three grown children who live across our great country, one grandson, and four fur babies. They are all the light of my life and my reason for being. We have been very fortunate to have a loving family who love and support us and who we love back and are very proud of.

This book is not about the pandemic nor the changes our world has undertaken, so let's just be clear about that. I don't care what your vaccine status is or if you believe in vaccines; I don't care about that. Your choice, your right. But I digress, back to the purpose of this book. The purpose is to look at my, or rather *our*, transition from being healthcare workers to being a patient, who is now a COVID long hauler and the spouse of a patient, as well as our restored faith in God. Our journey through this terrifying experience has been life changing, some good changes and some not so good.

During our thirty-six years of marriage, we have overcome many obstacles, including my husband's many deployments as a Chief Hospital Corpsman in the United States Navy. He was gone quite frequently during illnesses and deaths of family members. We experienced the death of parents together, but one of the toughest to overcome was my being in the hospital when my husband was not allowed to visit me. The not knowing *if* I would ever come home was excruciating for him and our family. And let me not forget to mention, it wasn't a vacation for me either. It wasn't like I went away on a girl's trip to the spa. I wasn't on a pampering trip, that's for sure!

This book is about our journey through a terrifying ordeal called COVID-19 that could very well have taken my life and the changes that have happened over the last almost-three years. The real-life miracle that occurred during a pandemic, when the world was going crazy, the ongoing complications of COVID-19 and the Long Covid syndrome have brought some very permanent changes to our lives. Throughout our journey, one thing became clear—God is definitely in control! I am living proof of the miracles only God can do. By all accounts, I should not be sitting here today writing this book. The odds were stacked against me. The medical professionals had already written me off as a goner.

What I experienced was nothing short of one of God's miracles and proof that He really is the conductor of this orchestra known as life and ultimately, the world. We hear these stories all the time. How Bobby Jo experienced a miracle; how John Smith experienced a miracle after a car crash, and so on, but this book is our account of a special miracle that not only saved my life but changed our lives for the better. It's about how our God is truly the God of Ephesians 3:20 (NIV)

> *Now to Him who is able to do immeasurably more than all we ask or imagine according to His power that is at work within us.*

At first it was hard to believe that we were able to begin writing this book and that God had commissioned me to do this. The thought He has instilled in my heart is that if I can help just one person navigate their journey through COVID or Long COVID, then His miracle was well worth it. He wanted me to share our story through one of the worst experiences we have ever been through—and not only share our story, but also to help those who are struggling with something in their life, giving others hope that there is a greater Power to turn to. I know there are others out there experiencing Long COVID; I know they are feeling like freaks of nature just like me, and this book will hopefully give them some encouragement not to rely solely on themselves, but to lean on God and follow His direction for their lives. We certainly do not feel like subject-matter experts on COVID, the Bible, or even life itself. But here we are. We are just ordinary folks trying to be obedient

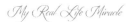

with a calling that God has placed on our hearts. We hope you will enjoy and perhaps even learn something about yourself while on this journey with us. We certainly have learned a lot in the last three years.

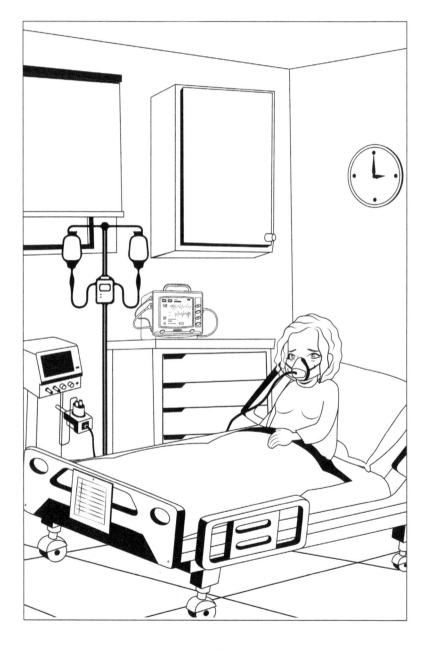

The Beginning

When, exactly was the beginning? Every story has a beginning, but when was mine? Was it the end of 2019 when the first cases of COVID-19 were being diagnosed in Wuhan, China? Or, was it in March 2020 when then-President Trump put the whole country on a fourteen-day lockdown? Remember that? Just fourteen days to stop the spread? We all know how well that worked out. Or was it before that? Was it a combination of wrong turns along the way? That has yet to be determined, and quite honestly, I have my own opinion on when the beginning was, but we will talk about that later in another chapter.

Let me set the stage so you can begin to form your own opinion. Grab a cup of coffee, sit back, and relax. Let's get started.

Some would say the beginning is before birth. God knows exactly when you will be conceived, to whom and where you would be born, and on which day. Some would say the cycle of life began way before you were even a twinkle in the eyes of your parents or their parents and so forth. Some say every life began with Adam and Eve. We are all God's children. He is our Father in heaven. He provides for us. He knows the plans for our lives. He is the conductor of the orchestra known as life.

We seem to be pawns on the celestial chess board, moving around as we are directed to by a much higher Power. Yes, we have minds and oftentimes make the wrong decisions in our lives, and yes, we take the wrong turns—more than once, I am sure. Some of us more than others, especially me. I never was good at following directions. We were given minds and the ability to make choices. Some of us make better choices than others but the choice is ours, just the same. And then you live with the consequences. Yes, we each wear many different hats, and we have different titles but none more important than to be known as God's obedient servants. But are we obedient 100 percent of the time? Be honest. If you need to, this is a good time to put this book down, grab that cup of coffee, and do some self-reflection. I will be here when you get back. I'm not going anywhere. Thankfully, I have lots of time.

I am no different. I've done that self-reflection. You may not like what you see. I didn't like everything I saw. And yes, I recognized the need for change.

I, like so many others, have many titles: wife, mom, memaw, daughter, sister, aunt, and cousin; but my favorite title is being known as a daughter of Christ, our God who only wants good for His children. He is a God that loves me unconditionally, no matter how many times I screw up. Trust me, that has been a lot! Actually, one title I probably wear very well is that of professional screwup! God knows what is best and has the most perfect plan for our lives. Doesn't that just give you warm fuzzies all over? Don't you just feel safe and secure, knowing that our God has the best plans for us, no matter how much or how bad we mess up? No matter how many times we make stupid mistakes, He is there to forgive us. He created us in His image, and all we have to do is know He loves us and live accordingly. You see, God knows what will happen in your life before you do. One of my favorite Bible verses, Jeremiah 29:11 (NIV) states:

> *"For I know the plans I have for you declares the Lord.*
> *Plans to prosper you and not to harm you, plans to give*
> *you hope and a future."*

According to this scripture, God knows the plans for you; He knows what will happen to you and exactly when. Don't you just love that? It doesn't mean that life will always be peaches and cream. Life won't and can't be seen through rose-colored glasses or lived through a filter. There will be good times and bad. There will be health and sickness, sadness, and happiness. There will be many ups and downs; trials and tribulations but hopefully lots of celebrations and love. While we know life involves all kinds of emotions and feelings, we always hope for more love and happiness. But we should also remember that God doesn't promise us just roses; there will be thorns along the way. It's what we do with those thorns that really show us how much grit and grace we have been given. In Genesis 50:20 (NIV) Joseph said:

> *"You intended to harm me but God intended it all for good, He brought me to this position so I could save the lives of many people."*

God had a plan to send His one and only Son, Jesus Christ, to offer us salvation and eternal life in heaven, living with the Father. He intended nothing but good for us. Even though we may experience pain and suffering, bad breaks, and all kinds of setbacks, He has a plan; and when these not-so-nice things happen to us, it is God's way of deterring us from the wrong path, slowing us down to match His perfect timing or just giving us a little detour so we will appreciate it all the more when we finally reach God's intended destiny for our lives.

Now that I have piqued your curiosity, let's start from the beginning. The beginning of my story was in November 2020. This was the month of our very own D-Day. My husband and I came down with symptoms about the same time; however, mine was just a sore throat, and I didn't think anything of it. My husband was not feeling well at all, and it was my job as the wife and nurse to care for my husband. It was a Sunday, so the next day, I made my husband get tested at work for COVID-19, although neither of us really expecting it to

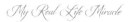

be positive. My husband always gets a cold this time of year, so we chalked it up to his yearly cold. But much to my dismay, he was positive, and I was beginning to feel worse with each passing day.

I went from having a slight sore throat to a cough and severe shortness of breath in what seemed like a blink of the eye. I was too busy to get sick. Who had time for a runny nose, sniffles, or coughing? Not this girl. I just put my hand up and said, "Ah, excuse me, talk to the hand, not today, Satan." Since my first test was negative, I was tested a second time because with my husband now positive, and my fever was worsening. It was hard to believe I was negative that first test. Lucky girl, right? Didn't I tell Satan to stay away? Well, he listened as well as a teenager with raging hormones.

My only severe symptoms at that time were a high fever and cough. After a few more days of battling through that, my fever broke, but my cough was getting worse. We thought we were in the clear, which meant we had the rest of the fourteen-day quarantine to rest and relax at home without a care in the world! Everything we have ever been taught in the medical field was once a fever breaks, you are on your way to recovery. We were already planning the many things we would spend our time doing: online Christmas shopping, binge-watching movies, eating lots of popcorn, and catching up on some much-needed sleep. You know, the usual things a married couple would do when quarantined together for fourteen days. Whoever expected to be quarantined for that long? Didn't that only happen in the movies? We were excited for some free staycation time! You know what they say about well laid-out plans. Ours soon was trashed. Our free staycation on the government's dime just went to hell in a handbasket. God must have thought I needed a wakeup call, and I was about to get the jolt of my life. A jolt much stronger than any coffee you could ever consume.

My symptoms started to progress from a fever to body aches, headaches, and congestion. Then suddenly, exactly one week after testing positive for COVID-19, I could not breathe; I mean I literally could not breathe. I had difficulty eating, showering, and brushing my teeth. Anything that required me to use oxygen suddenly became very difficult, and very scary. I sent my husband out to the store to get a portable pulse oximeter so I could see what my oxygen saturation was. When he returned home and placed it on my finger, it was in the eighties! I thought the stupid thing was broken! That was a waste of seventeen bucks! There was no way that was right because normal is above 96 percent.

Later that evening, after multiple readings and still no change, my husband took me to the emergency room. He walked me in, and when the nurse behind the desk noticed I could barely talk from being out of breath, she told me to have a seat behind the desk. My oxygen saturation was 65 percent! The emergency room nurse and I were completely shocked! I kissed my husband with tears running down my cheeks and noticed he was trying very hard to hold it together, but I knew he was scared, and I knew I was in trouble. We had both seen a lot of sickness and death in our thirty-plus years as medical professionals, but this involved us. Our thought was *This can't be.* Some think that medical experience is a benefit, but sometimes knowing can be a huge detriment. Visitors were not allowed during this time, so he walked out of the emergency room, head hung low, looking like a lost puppy who had lost his best friend and sat in the truck for what seemed liked hours.

He made the necessary family calls and then made the dreaded call to my dad. He knew that call was not going to be easy. We had already lost my mother a few years before, and that almost tore my dad apart. All of us in the family held him together. We each were a piece of the fragile puzzle that held him up.

After sitting in the parking lot of the emergency room for what seemed like hours, he finally made the drive home after I promised him that I would be alright and that I would be home by Sunday. No way was I staying in the hospital longer than a day or two and no way was I missing Thanksgiving with my family. After I let him know, I was safely in my hospital room, he finally went home. His head down, feeling defeated and lost. It killed me to hear the sound of such utter defeat in his voice. That was the first of many more times that I would hear that. It broke my heart each time and each time, it strengthened my resolve to make it home to my family. Remember the saying, "when the going gets tough, the tough get going". Well, that kept going on in my head as if on a loop. Over and over again.

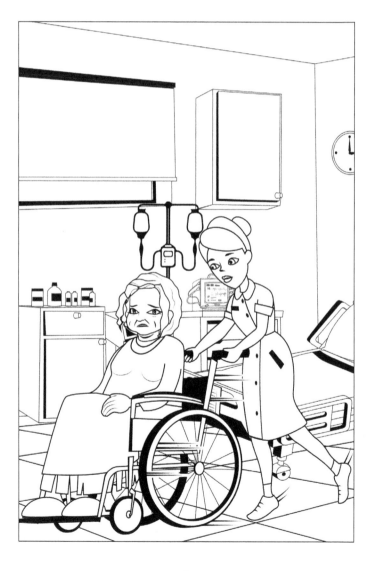

The triage nurse called some kind of special code, one I am sure meant, "I'm coming in hot with another COVID'er," over her walkie talkie and whisked me into the back at a pace that seemed like she was running at warped speed. When she got me into the ER room, I noticed they were set up for an intubation. I knew what that meant. I recognized the tools and the setup because I had been the one to set it up too many times, but this was the first time being on this side of the situation. This was a side I was not liking at all; being a patient instead of the nurse sucked. I knew what was going on, and I recognized all the signs. It added up to me being in serious trouble.

It was the first time it hit me that I was really, seriously sick, not just sick but critically ill. I felt this overwhelming sense of hatred at this moment. I truly hated COVID-19 and what this was going to put my family through—right before Thanksgiving and right before what would be another of my mother's heavenly birthdays. Who was going to take care of my husband and son while I was in the hospital? Who was doing the laundry, cooking, and being the peacekeeper? I know they were adults; but let's face it, they rely on Mom.

The ER doctor came in and halted everything. He put me on a non-rebreather mask and told everyone to hold on and see what my oxygen saturation (sats) was after giving me oxygen. My SATS immediately responded and went to 97 percent! *Thank you, God!* No ventilator for me—At least not right now! After a while, they took the non-rebreather off and put me on a nasal cannula, and my sats held steady. The normal ER song and dance occurred, you know, the usual blood work, an IV was started and the chest x-ray was performed. Dr. Smith came in to show my films to me and explain that I had the infamous "ground glass clutter" that indicated COVID-19 pneumonia. My lungs were bad, he told me. I was in for a long haul of treatments and recovery, but he sounded optimistic. He even mentioned the possibility of sending me home on oxygen because the number of COVID patients admitted had left the hospital, with few free beds remaining. I thought, *Somehow, I couldn't get that lucky.*

I was admitted to the COVID ward for the next several days or a week, I can't remember exactly how long. The next day when the doctor came in to see me, he started the typical COVID-19 protocol. I was started on antibiotics, given a three-day course of Remdesivir and one plasma treatment. I continued to get worse over the course of several days. My husband was home and had access to my online chart, so he was following my lab results, and chest x-rays and numerous CT scans to rule out a pulmonary embolus (blot clot in my lungs). He was not liking what he was seeing and began to become more and more concerned.

We could not talk, but I could tell how worried he was by his text messages. We tried to have a brief conversation every morning and night, but talking made my coughing and breathing worse. I lost track of time. Days turned into nights and nights into days. I was still on oxygen but just a nasal cannula and then eventually high-flow oxygen. I felt like I was in prison.

Around Thanksgiving, the doctors began to ask me every day if I would sign a "Do Not Resuscitate (DNR)" order, and every day, I refused. Did they really think I would sign a piece of paper stating I didn't want any lifesaving interventions? Did they really believe I had no reason to want to survive? I really felt like they wanted me to sign the DNR, be put on the ventilator so they could push the hospital bed into a dark corner somewhere and leave me there until I died. The nurse in me knows that couldn't possibly be true, but the patient in me really felt so. They wanted to put me on BIPAP (bi-level positive airway pressure) mask, but I refused. Even though I knew this positive-pressure mask would help get much needed oxygen into my lungs faster and better than a regular nasal cannula or even the high flow oxygen but doing so, I knew that would be one step closer to being put on a ventilator, and somehow, I just knew the ventilator was not for me. I couldn't explain it at the time, but now I know that God was telling me to refuse it. I literally felt if I was placed on the ventilator that would be a death sentence, but God was telling me to fight and to have faith. So, I did. I didn't realize at the time where that strong conviction to refuse was coming from, but I eventually figured it out. Stay tuned.

This entire time I was afraid to go to sleep because I knew I was hypoxic (low oxygen levels in your blood), and I was afraid the doctors would sedate me and put me on a ventilator without my knowledge. As a nurse, I knew they could not legally do that without my consent, but I worried they would call my husband, and since we could not talk on the phone, he would not know what was going on and consent for me. Keep in mind, during this time, family members were not allowed in the hospital at all. One of the smartest things my husband did before taking me to the hospital was put my cell phone charger in my purse so I was able to keep my phone charged so we could text. That was the only form of communication we had. Talking made me cough, and coughing made me short of breath. It was a never-ending cycle. I could not lay completely down in the bed, so I sat up, leaning forward for hours at times because I was having so much difficulty catching my breath. It felt like a lifetime since I had laid flat in the bed or was able to breathe—but it had only been a week.

The day after Thanksgiving, my breathing got worse. I knew I was heading in the wrong direction, and my health was going down the toilet. The doctor once again asked me to go on BIPAP, and once again, I refused. He asked me to sign a DNR, and once again, I refused. He left the room scratching his head. He ordered a chest CT scan to rule out a pulmonary embolism again. The nurse, Janice, and respiratory therapist, Annette, assigned to me on this day were two of the worst in their respective professions that I had ever seen. My IV needed to be changed prior to them taking me to CT. Janice started it, attempted to flush it, and I told her it was not a good line. I felt it infiltrating but she blew me off and stated it was fine. I knew otherwise.

After several hours, they were ready to take me to CT. They packaged me up and off we went. They ran into several walls with the hospital bed and had difficulty getting it in the elevator, and I thought

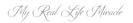

to myself, *Oh, God, they are going to kill me!* We finally made it to CT, and the techs took over. Once they got me in the CT room and moved me onto the CT table, Janice and Annette left the room. The two techs asked me if I was okay because I guess I must have looked terrified. I told them they were horrible drivers and kept running me into walls on the way down there!

I laugh about it now, and trust me, I know it isn't easy to steer a stretcher, but this was like a comedy act! I had two people who did not seem competent caring for me! I mean, there were so many hospital employees who stopped and asked them if they needed help, but of course, they said they didn't. It seemed like they were having just a grand ole time at my expense. Just picture it, Dumb and Dumber in those ruffled old-time tuxedos trying to steer a hospital bed down hospital corridors. It makes you want to laugh at the picture it gives you and cry at the same time! What a nightmare!

The techs, of course, had to restart my IV because the one Janice started was in fact, infiltrated. After the scan was completed, the comedy act continued as I headed back. Once in my room, the nursing assistant, Sally, sat next to my bed, holding my hand and asking me if I was okay because I was shaking and out of breath. That night was the worse night yet, and in spite of all that, it was also the best. See, I had two heavenly visitors that night in my hospital room. Afterward, I consented to being put in a CPAP mask because I really could not breathe. It was at that moment in time when I had those two visitors that I knew, really knew, that I was going to be okay—I was not going to die.

The doctor came in very early the next morning and asked me again about going on BIPAP, and this time, I consented. I think I repeated it more than once because he couldn't believe what he was hearing. He informed me I was being transferred to the ICU. The ICU physician on duty came to see me in the COVID unit. She told me that if I needed to be on BIPAP for a long time, they would need to intubate me and put me on the ventilator. I was determined that was not going to happen because my late-night visitors assured me it would not. They told me I would be okay, so I was at peace and knew I would never need the ventilator. Maybe my two visitors were figments of my imagination? Maybe they were from an extreme hypoxic event, or perhaps I had just gone completely crazy and was hallucinating. We will let you decide later.

They put me on BIPAP, and I was transferred to the ICU. I was once again asked to sign a DNR, which I refused once again. Little did I know that after seeing me, the ICU physician called my husband at 7 a.m., informing him that I was on BIPAP and headed to the ICU. She also informed him that I was minutes away from being put on the ventilator, and if I was, I would never come off of it. He should prepare for the worst-case scenario—that I was going to die. She also asked him to make me a DNR, but he refused. The impression was given that I was going to be in the ICU for a very long time or until I did die.

As I am writing this, it strikes me again just how very lucky I am to be here typing this today, almost two in a half years later. It gives me chills and brings tears to my eyes even now. I am so very thankful for my second chance.

I was on BIPAP for almost thirty-six hours, but it felt like a lifetime. I had a central line placed, and it was discovered I had a deep vein thrombosis (DVT), a blood clot, behind my left knee. That was a total shocker as I had no symptoms except shortness of breath, but then again, my lungs were covered with the infamous ground-glass clutter of COVID pneumonia, so shortness of breath was expected! After quite some time, I was taken off the BIPAP so I could eat something and see how my O_2 sats did. Well, they stayed up above 88 percent! I did a little victory dance—well, in my head anyway! In fact, they held steady at about 90–92 percent. I stayed off BIPAP and on the high flow oxygen all night, and into the next day, I was still holding steady. I was still critical but improving.

I was in the ICU for three days until they needed the ICU bed for yet another critical COVID patient. They transferred me to the CCU Step-Down Unit in the middle of the night. I continued to improve in the CCU and was able to take two steps from the bed to the chair

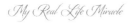

and back. I had forgotten what it felt like to stand on my own two feet! What an amazing feeling, even if it sent my breathing into a tailspin! I can't remember how many days I had been hospitalized at this point, but I just knew it was a step in the right direction. I was still on high-flow oxygen and waiting not so patiently for the respiratory therapist to begin weaning me off. I was in the CCU for over a week and never got the high-flow oxygen turned down! I had another week before I was determined to be home. I wanted to be home before my birthday and to see my son off to his dream job across the country.

One afternoon, my nurse suggested I FaceTime with my husband since it had been so long since I had seen him. He told me I was looking very good that particular day and that my husband would love to see me looking so well. I took his advice and dialed up FaceTime. I was in total shock how I looked! I looked nothing like myself. In fact, I didn't recognize myself. If he thought I looked particularly good on this day, what in the world did I look like yesterday? I was always the type who was in full makeup and hair done before ever leaving my house. No one *ever* saw me without full makeup on. My hair might have been pulled up on my head, but my makeup was on point. I even wore makeup when I went to CrossFit. Not that it was still on when I got done, but I least showed up with it on.

Before I could hang up, my husband answered, and the love and joy on his face took away any misgivings I had about my appearance. We chatted for a few minutes before the coughing took over again, but it was *so good* to see his face. I stayed in the CCU for a week or so longer until they came to me late one afternoon and told me they needed my room for another patient. Out of all the units I had been on, this was the only one where I didn't feel like I was in prison or more appropriately, a prisoner in isolation. I was being transferred back to the COVID unit where I had started. I was sad and depressed. I did not want to go back there, as I had horrifying memories of when I went into the hospital. My concerns fell on deaf ears. The bed was needed for someone much sicker than I was, although it was a bittersweet pill to swallow. I was glad I was being considered "not that sick," but I was also terrified of going back to where it all began. What was I going to do if that nurse on that dreadful day was assigned to me again? Time to put my big girl pants on and remember the nurse that I am. Alas, to my dread, I was transferred back later that evening.

I was determined I was not going backward. These nurses had too many patients to care for and were exhausted. I was determined I would continue to improve, with or without them. It seemed I was continuing to learn patience and gratitude as I was forced to wait for Respiratory Therapy to wean me off the high-flow oxygen. I could not go home until I was off the high-flow oxygen. The waiting was so very frustrating! I still only got out of the bed to take two steps to the chair and back. I had not walked since I walked into the emergency room on that first nightmarish night days ago or was it weeks? I could not get out of bed without help. I was totally dependent upon the staff. It was so frustrating for an independent woman to *wait* on everyone else for help! It was a humbling and valuable life lesson. Days turned into nights, and nights turned into days and still I waited to be weaned off the high-flow oxygen. I even looked it up on YouTube how to do it myself! The problem was, I could not reach it without help, and that was not going to happen!

The weekend was approaching, and I wanted so badly to go home. The physician, caring for me, told me on Friday morning that I had to do a six-minute walk test before he could discharge me home with oxygen, and he gently reminded me I also needed to be off the high-flow oxygen. Again, he spoke to the respiratory therapist who once again ignored the orders and did not wean me. At 4 p.m. that afternoon, the therapist came in, whipped the high-flow oxygen off me, set a walker in front of me, and told me to get up and walk around my hospital room. I asked her if she was going to put a nasal cannula on me, and she stated, "No, get up and walk." I stood up and took two steps. My O$_2$ sats plummeted into the toilet. Where was the empathy? Where was the care and compassion?

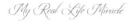

I was made to sit down, and the high flow put back on me. She told me that she knew I couldn't do it. At this point, I was angry and frustrated, and with tears streaming down my face, I asked her what did she expect? I know I mentioned that I had not walked since walking into the emergency room, and I had been on oxygen since that dreadful night. I still wonder to this day, what exactly did she expect someone in my condition to do? I was furious at the audacity of her treating me and other patients like this. She didn't care and had no empathy for my situation. I could not believe the lack of caring she had displayed. What had the healthcare profession come to? It was one more reason to hate COVID-19. It had hardened almost everyone's heart toward the real plight of patients.

As a healthcare worker myself, this was hard for me to comprehend. I knew the staff was overworked, had way too many patients, and this virus was still so new that we were learning on the go, but to be completely unempathetic was just something I could not fathom. I was livid. My nurse came into the room and saw me crying. She helped me back into the bed, and when I told her, she couldn't believe what had happened. She stormed out to speak with the charge nurse. After several minutes, she stormed back in with a nasal cannula, furious herself. She stated that the charge nurse informed her to put me on a nasal cannula at six liters, and when my sats nosedived again, that would shut me up.

It was just so unbelievable, another unempathetic healthcare worker. She looked me right in the eyes and told me she knew I could do it and said a quick prayer with me. She became my very own cheerleader! Off with the high-flow oxygen mask and on went the nasal cannula. My sats stayed steady at 90 percent! We did it! I was off the High Flow Oxygen! I was so proud of myself—and so terrified at the same time! The entire night, despite encouragement from the night respiratory therapist, I played the "what if" game in my head.

I was afraid my sats would drop.

I was afraid to go backward.

I was afraid I would find myself in the ICU again.

I was just afraid.

Terrified, actually, and stressed.

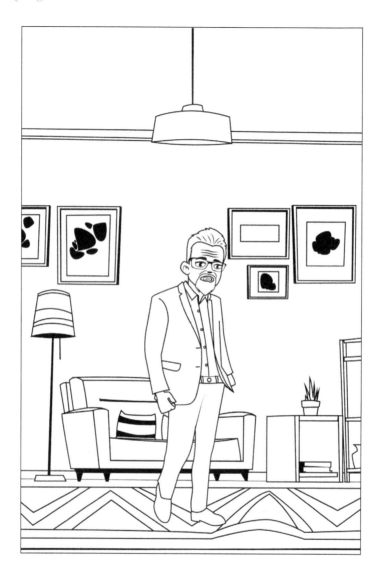

Reflections from David

What have I done? I did this. I brought this home to our house, and I am the one responsible. I got my wife, my best friend, the most important person in my world, critically sick. She became sick on Monday, one week after I became sick and tested positive for COVID-19. She took care of me for that first week, and I was feeling much better. But now, Lisa was sick and had a fever for three days. She was feeling bad but nothing extreme. We really thought that if we could control or get rid of this fever, everything would be okay. Afterall, isn't that the goal with almost every illness: beat the fever? Control the fever and things improve and then recovery? But COVID-19 wasn't every other illness. We were able to break the fever by day three and thought we had it licked. Day four started with Lisa having a lot of difficulty breathing and catching her breath. It didn't matter what position she tried; she was having breathing issues. That entire day she did nothing but sleep. For the next two days, she attempted to get comfortable but just couldn't.

Her breathing was not improving at all. I went to the store and bought a pulse oximeter to check her O_2 saturation. When I got home, I had her put it on her finger, and her oxygen sats were in the 80s initially but kept getting worse throughout the day.

On Friday, two days post-fever, she was really getting worse. I asked her if she wanted to go to the hospital, and she said no way. I kept watching her, and she looked worse and worse. Finally, at 8

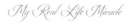

o'clock that evening, I told her that she was going to the hospital. She agreed.

I was scared to death, and I could see it in her eyes that she was too. Sometimes it is a blessing to have a medical background because you can anticipate what is going to happen, but this COVID-19 virus was different. Nobody, not even the doctors, knew exactly what or how to treat it successfully. Treatment had been a trial-by-error approach. I had COVID, so I knew I wasn't going to be able to stay with her. I made sure that she had her cellphone charger with her in her purse. This will prove to be one of the smartest things I could have done.

We drove the fifteen minutes to the hospital, a quiet drive because again, being healthcare providers, we knew that this was going to be difficult. Once at the hospital, we walked slowly from the truck (she was having difficulty walking and breathing) in the front doors of the emergency department. They took her right back to the triage area and told me that I had to go outside. I was only in my truck for two or three minutes when Lisa called to tell me they were admitting her to the COVID floor ASAP. Her oxygen sats were only 66 at check in.

We knew from the news stories that people with COVID were being put on ventilators, and most often they were not coming off of them. Lisa said even before we went to the hospital that she would never be put on a ventilator. I was scared. My thoughts were everywhere. Was this really happening to us? To her? Did I wait too long to take her to the hospital? Was that the last time I was going to see my wife? Whatever happened to being able to advocate for your loved ones when they can't advocate for themselves? I just knew that this was going to be a huge uphill battle. Was this all my fault?

She told me that I should just go home for the night because since I wasn't allowed in the hospital, there was nothing I could do. I knew that, but that was my wife of thirty-four years, my soulmate and best friend. How could I be made to leave her at the very moment of our lives when she needed me the most?

I drove back home slowly, and during this drive is when I reached out and placed my faith in God. We are Christians, but we had a bad experience with a church seventeen years prior and hadn't been back since. I told God that I was sorry for abandoning Him for as long as I had, but I truly needed Him to forgive me and asked Him to please give my wife the strength that she needed to battle this virus and come home. "Please protect and heal my wife."

I had to go home and tell my children, my father-in-law and my mother what was happening. I knew that they were all going to have a million questions, but at this point, I just didn't have any answers. My mother and my father-in-law were the only ones who truly knew what was going on in my mind and heart; you see, each had lost their spouses over the last few years. The only person I could truly reach out to right now and the only one who could in fact bring her home was God.

I'm ashamed to say it but until that moment, I had never prayed that much with that much conviction in my entire life. I couldn't sleep, so there was nothing better to do but to pray and pray some more. It sounds a little crazy, but I could truly feel that the Lord was listening to me, and through prayer, I was somewhat at peace knowing that no matter what, He was in control.

Remember I told you earlier that one of the smartest things I did, besides pray, was to pack Lisa's cellphone charger in her purse? We spoke occasionally but texted each day. She was keeping me updated, and I was able to track her lab work and doctor's notes via a patient portal. We *never* ended a phone call without saying, "I love you"! Texting was also extremely important, and this allowed me to advocate for her as well as keep up with what the doctors were doing and thinking, based on the medications, labs, and x-rays that were being ordered.

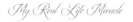

The Dreaded Day Seven

Friday evening, one week after being admitted, she was having increased difficulty breathing; the high-flow oxygen just wasn't working. She spent the first six days sitting straight up in bed. If she sat back, she couldn't catch her breath. In the middle of the night Friday night, the doctors decided they needed to transfer her to the ICU. The thought was that she was more than likely going to need to be placed on a ventilator. I spoke with her on the phone, but it was very difficult for her to communicate. I told her to save her breath, I love you, and to text me instead. I could tell that she was extremely scared, and I stepped up my praying more and more.

Day Eight—Saturday at 7 a.m.

My cellphone rang, and I saw it was the hospital. My heart sank and for a second stopped beating. It was the hospitalist taking care of Lisa. He said, "Good morning Mr. Amick." He told me who he was and asked me, "Have you considered making your wife a DNR because she is minutes away from needing to be placed on a venti-lator"? My exact words to him were, "Have you spoken to my wife about this? Because I don't think you know who you are dealing with."

Faith Tested

F aith. I have had a lot of time to reflect back on where my faith was
at that time. Yes, I had faith, but it had been tested. And if I am
honest with myself, I pushed it down deep inside me and didn't think
another thing about it. My anger was so great when my mother died
that I suppressed my faith. Faith without good deeds is dead faith,
isn't that what we are taught? Well, I guess there you have it. I had
dead faith. Okay, maybe not dead faith; it was there deep down inside
where I had buried it, never to surface again. I felt like a complete and
utter failure when my mother died. I had let everyone down. So, in
order to keep putting one foot in front of the other and pretending
to have my act together, I suppressed my faith. I buried it deep down
inside of me and refused to let even a glimpse of it out. The more I
buried it, the more my anger came to the surface. How was my faith
was tested? I know it was, and I failed the test.

I completely believe my faith journey could have begun with either
one of two life-altering events, both events truly testing me. The few
years before the COVID pandemic were full of ups and downs, trials
and tribulations, including a new job, the loss of two family members
that was absolutely devastating, and just your normal, everyday life
events that are rather boring.

Let's start with the most difficult experience I have ever gone
through, a most life-shattering event. Several years ago, in 2016, when
my mother became ill and was hospitalized. She was in the hospital
for a few months before passing away on August 26, 2016. At first,

no one was sure what was going on with her. She was confused, and her blood sugar was out of control even though she was a very knowledgeable and controlled diabetic. It was unstable one day and stable the next. It was a very bizarre hospital course. Bottom line, she ended up on a ventilator but was alert and oriented and able to communicate with us. She had a trach and was eventually transferred to a long-term rehab facility, where she continued to improve until she could be transferred to a short-term rehab when she started exhibiting signs of infection and was transferred to a well-known, major-medical facility. They were able to isolate the bacterium causing the infection, and she made drastic improvements.

She was doing so well until she wasn't.

It was a beautiful Sunday in August. We had such a great time in her hospital room that afternoon. We laughed a lot. It was the first time in three months that I heard her call me by my name. She sat up in that bed, wiggling her little feet, still with a trach but breathing on her own and not having any difficulty talking to us. We had so much fun. I don't think I had ever laughed so hard. We left a little early because she was having surgery in the morning. You see, the infection had eaten away at her spine, and they were going in to fix it. She had gotten that strong the past few weeks. We were already making plans for the day she came home from the hospital. We would have a huge family gathering with lots of food and laughter. I stood outside that room, hesitating to leave; my feet just didn't want to move. It was the great day we had, or perhaps I wanted to stay and continue catching up or maybe something else was bothering me.

But I left. I just turned and walked away, not knowing I would never see her smile at me again.

At 4 AM, the phone rang, and I remember hearing my dad yell for me to pick up the phone. It was the hospital. My mom had choked on a mucous plug and coded. They had to do CPR on her and had no idea how long she was down before they found her. Five days later, my mother passed away. I kept thinking that I should have stayed with her that night, that maybe if I had been there, she would still be here. I'm a nurse. I know to listen to my instincts, but I didn't. I failed my mother, my father, my brother; I failed my entire family. My parents were like peanut butter and jelly. Good ole PB&J, and I let them down. I never did figure out which one was the peanut butter and which one was the jelly, but I like to think they were each a little bit of both. My dad would say my mom was the glue that held us together, but I think it was both of them. And I let them down—I let everyone down. What kind of nurse was I anyway? What kind of daughter was I? I was almost done with my doctorate in nursing, but how could I continue? I was left wondering what kind of nurse I was. A failure, a complete, utter failure. That's what I was. I became angry at myself. I was a terrible daughter and sister—a complete failure. I didn't deserve to be a nurse. I didn't deserve my family. This was a heavy burden I would carry for a long time.

Why on earth was I a nurse when I could not save my own mother? Everyone looked to me for answers, and I just didn't have any; I was at a complete loss. Then I became angry with God. Why did He put her, us, through all this? Why did He give us such a great day and then take her away like that? Why? I seriously questioned my faith, questioning everything, and I was quickly losing hope and faith. No, I lost complete faith in everything, including God. I was still so wrapped up in my grief and anger that one day in November after my mother passed away, I was in the bathroom talking to my mother-in-law and sister-in-law while they were doing hair and makeup for my nephew's wedding that evening. They were giggling and carrying on like mothers and daughters do and I just quietly walked out without so much as a word to anyone to wallow in my grief. To this day, I do not think either of them realized I was fighting back tears when I left the room. I'm not sure how long it took them to realize I had snuck out of the bathroom.

Eventually, God led people into my life that helped me realize that I could not control any of the events that led up to my mother's death.

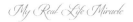

God has a plan, and everything happens according to His plan in His perfect timing. That perfect last day we had with her? It was part of God's plan so we would have those memories to cling to. Great memories. Those memories are far better than if we only had the ones of her on the ventilator. Even though I had come to terms with that, I still realize that my career was spiraling out of control. I had just transferred my grief and anger to my job and ambitions. I was heading into uncharted territory. I had ignored what God was telling me to do. I had professional goals, and whether I achieved those goals were in my control—or at least, that is what I told myself. I had plans of my own for my career, and I was bound and determined to accomplish them.

The second event began a few months before I actually tested positive for COVID-19 and certainly before I went in the hospital. It began with my *job*. The stress I had been under at work had increased significantly the year prior to my illness. In fact, just let me be completely transparent, I was not in a good place. I had taken a detail into another position to get away from a hostile environment I had been in. The hostility never went away even though I was in a different position, but rather, it intensified. I was stressed, very unhappy at my situation, and to top things off, I was being kicked out of my office. I know that is a minor inconvenience, but at the time to me, it was a major deterrence. My office was in boxes scattered all over the place and in the trunk of my government vehicle, which was adding to my stress. I was leading so many projects, and now I did not know where any of my reference materials were. I was basically homeless and living out of my government vehicle. I just could not function like that. I had no idea how I was going to continue in this manner and be effective in my detailed position. The icing on the cake, was the person hired for the position I had been doing had been onboard for a couple of months now and completely had the con. He did not need me. I really had no job, and yet I was being forced to stay in a double-encumbered position, and it was just not a place anyone wants to be in. I was flying by the seat of my pants, with no real authority and no real job. He did not need me; no one needed me. I felt useless. I began to function more in the role of a clinical consultant for him and nursing expert for the nursing staff. I was going down a path God did not want me to follow, but I was not listening. I marched on, ignoring the signs, and trust me, there were many. Even though I had no idea where I was going or what my next move was, I was in a nonexistent job, with no direction and no future at this point. But I still marched forward with blinders on.

Believe me, there were a lot of signs.

But. I. Ignored. Every. One. Of. Them.

You see, I was so wrapped up in my own despair and stress that I did not see the signs that God was trying to use to get my attention. I had ignored His gentle nudges. The feathers and pennies that were suddenly in my path were ignored. The beautiful butterflies I saw were ignored, and even the cardinals seen in my backyard were ignored. All signs from God were ignored. I did not listen to that whispered voice in my head, telling me this was not the plan; those urges put on my heart or even the messages from God in the form of devotionals were ignored. I was a hot mess! What was worse, I was a hot mess of my own making. No one else was to blame for my current state of being—just me. My heart, my eyes, and my ears were closed off, and I could not see what was right in front of me. All I saw was where I wanted to be but had no clue how to get there.

I had been a nurse for a very long time, and this was the first time in my career that I felt completely and totally lost. I didn't feel like I belonged in my job, I didn't belong in the detailed job, and I certainly did not belong at the facility I was working at. I was miserable professionally but knew I had a few more years to go before I reached my retirement. I was not sure if I was going to make it, so I was trying to figure out my next move. I was trying to figure it out without God, without listening to Him. I was doing it on my own. Big mistake.

It was there the whole time.

So, what happens when you ignore God? Well, He gets your attention one way or another.

Numbers 22:28, 31 (NIV) states:

> *Then the Lord opened the donkey's mouth and she said to Balaam, what have I done to you to make you beat me these three times?... Then the Lord opened Balaam's eyes and he saw the angel of the Lord standing in the road with his sword drawn.*

When you don't listen to God, He gets your attention in any manner He can. In my case, I was headed down a path He did not want. In this verse, God used a donkey to speak. In my example, I got very sick. I got COVID-19 badly, I almost died and then during those lonely nights, isolated from everyone I loved and fearful I would die, God had my full attention. Stress can cause so many different health ailments, so many different emotions. Stress is a deterrent to listening to God. Self-ambition is a deterrent to listening to God, and so can grief. It can cause you to get inside your own head, and you can dig in so deep that it is hard to get out, even if someone throws you a life vest.

That was my first mistake.

Probably the biggest mistake of my life,

One that almost cost me my life.

But God wasn't done with me yet.

He had plans.

Several years before all this went down, we had been attending a church in our town. We were involved in our church's activities,

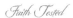

and our youngest son was very involved in the youth group. In fact, he even gave a sermon on Mother's Day. We did not miss a church service. I even sang in the choir. I know, right? Me! I sang in the church choir. It was at this church where my husband and I were baptized and accepted Jesus as our Lord and Savior. Even our youngest was baptized at this church. We stopped going because we discovered our pastor was more of a fraud than a true man of God. There were too many cliques and too much gossip mongers in this church. And if I am being honest, I never really felt close to God at this church. I didn't feel His presence. I really didn't have that intimate relationship with Him that I do now.

I know that all sounds a little weird but looking back, and hindsight is 20–20 after all; at the time, I didn't know what didn't feel right, but I never felt the presence of God the way I do now at church. The church we attend now is the same church. It has just been literally rebuilt, the pastor is new, and the members are all different. The virus that plagued the church the first time we attended it is long gone. The name and address are the same, but everything else is different. I feel God's presence in this church now. He is there every Sunday. My faith is not hidden anymore, and I wear it proudly and talk about it all the time with anyone and everyone who will listen and even a few that don't listen. I have that intimate relationship now that I have craved for so long. I hear God speak to me through diving into His word and I feel the Holy Spirit's presence in my heart. I feel the conviction of the Holy Spirit.

My Faith-filled Miracle

My faith went from being buried to being worn as a proud badge of honor. My life before getting sick was filled with ambition and self-proclaimed goals. I never realized it before, but my goals were just that, *my* goals. My life was busy. Our lives were busy. We never really thought about just how crazy our lives had gotten until quite some time after I came home. My experience was almost like that of the Grinch whose heart grew ten sizes. You could say my faith grew ten sizes as I experienced something magical, something miraculous.

In my dark room alone, I experienced my own little faith-filled miracle that was so magical and so life-changing. I will never forget how I felt that night. How my faith and confidence grew. How I just knew that something huge was coming. Something extraordinary was going to happen. The Bible mentions twenty-three accounts of miracles Jesus performed. Healing miracles, and the one common denominator of all those people was faith in God. They each believed and had complete faith in God. They did not need to see Him or need proof He was there. Every single person Jesus healed had faith. They were true believers.

There are many references in the Bible to the miracles that Jesus Christ performed. He healed the blind and the paralyzed, and He turned water into wine as well as helped fisherman with the biggest catch of fish in the history of fishing. In modern times, you hear of people who should not have survived a terrible health scare, walked away unscathed from an accident, and woke up from comas months later, even though the medical professionals never thought it possible. I experienced one of these myself.

The doctors treating me told my husband many times that I was not going to make it. They asked me to sign a DNR several times a day. My husband was told I was minutes away from going on the ventilator, and if that happened, I would not survive. In fact, no one expected me to survive.

I know it is very strange, even though I was scared, I never doubted that I was coming home.

Let me say that again, I never doubted I was coming home. I knew deep down I was coming home. I just knew. But how did I know?

I always knew I was going to live. I was astonished when asked to sign a DNR. Didn't they know I was going to be okay? I could not explain it at the time, but I knew I was going to live. Don't get me wrong, I was scared but something inside me just told me I was going to live.

One night after a very bad day, I was experiencing what I can only describe as a hypoxic anxiety attack. My heart was racing, and I was gasping for breath sitting up in the bed, grabbing the siderails so tight my knuckles were turning white. I kept watching the monitor as my heart rate went higher and higher and my oxygen saturation went lower and lower. The annoying alarms were causing my anxiety to increase and my headache to worsen. Quite honestly, I am sure it contributed significantly to everything that transpired that night. Of course, the nurses ignored the alarms, which drove me insane. Thinking back, all these episodes together in perfect harmony were creating the perfect storm for what was about to happen in the middle of that terrible night as I was sitting up in bed, feeling so very alone and helpless. My monitors were beeping, the IVAC machine was beeping. I could see them peeping in at me through that small window by the door yet not one person came in the room. I felt like I was in the middle of a terrible nightmare. It just wouldn't stop.

I was shaking uncontrollably.

I was scared.

No, let me rephrase that.

I was absolutely terrified.

I wanted so badly to call my husband, but I didn't want to worry him more than he already was. What was I going to say anyway? That I was

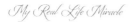

losing my mind? I had never in my life been so afraid, not even when my mother died and not even when my father-in-law died. Never in my life had I ever felt so very alone. *Not ever. Never ever, ever.*

I was isolated from my family and from the nursing staff. They came in, did whatever they needed to do, and hurried out of the room. The isolation was so deafening. I wish I could explain the feeling of complete, absolute loneliness, but I would never be able to explain it and give it justice. The only person who really held a conversation with me was the cleaning lady when she came in to empty the trash and sweep the floor every morning. She was a bright ray of sunshine. I looked forward to her visit every day. I had so much time on my hands to wonder, think, and pray. After all, you can only watch so many Hallmark Christmas movies. So, why did this happen to me? That was the million-dollar question going through my head as if on a loop, over and over again. *God chose me. He has plans for me. Then why was this happening to me?*

Writing this book is one example of His plans. I never would have thought about writing a book without Him. God wanted me to write this book and share my experience with whoever decided to read it or needed to read it. He wanted me to share how my faith was tested and how my faith grew. God used the spirits of my mother and father-in-law to comfort me. They were my angels that night. I know that they were only there for a few seconds, but it felt like a lifetime. I held onto that the rest of my hospital stay, and yes, I know my brain lacked oxygen at that point. I don't care. I know what I experienced, and it is my truth. I had never experienced anything like that before, and it was a feeling I never want to forget. I literally felt my mother's hand on my left hand. She just smiled at me and held my hand. My father-in-law stood up against that wall looking at me as he was willing his strength into me.

There are so many stories of people experiencing angel sightings, especially in life-and-death situations such as this. Mine was so life-changing, and the comfort it gave me is something I could never describe. I believe these special angels were sent to me for just that reason. They came to comfort and reassured me but also to let me know what I needed to do to get better. Even more so, they came to instill a deeper faith and understanding in God. As I would discover later, God had plans for me—big plans.

Yes, the news about COVID was terrifying. So many people were dying. But I knew I was not going to die. I was isolated from my family. I was alone, but I felt my perfect angels with me in that room, and it gave me hope as my faith continued to grow. I know the nurses were scared and overworked. They were exhausted. But I didn't let it put a damper in my newfound faith.

Having faith is imperative. Belief in what the Father is telling you is imperative. Jesus tells us many times that you must have faith and believe in what you cannot see, hear, or touch. Even if you only have a mustard seed of faith. Just because you can't see it, it doesn't mean it is not there. Your faith and belief should be there even when the circumstances of your life look bleak. And at this moment in time, my circumstances were very bleak. Faith and belief are what will carry you through the times when you are being tested. Put your blinders on and don't pay any attention to what the devil and his evil spirits are trying to tell you.

You can't just say you have faith without doing the deeds to support it. It's like telling everyone you are a Christian, yet you curse like a sailor. You shouldn't have to tell people you are a Christian; they should see it in your eyes and in your actions. Faith and belief go together like peanut butter and jelly. You can't have one without the other. In fact, you could say that it takes a sun-stand-still kind of faith and belief in today's world. That child-like innocence and trust is what God is expecting.

That is where the sun-stand-still faith and belief comes from. Look down deep and see if you can find the child inside of you. It's there; you just have to look deep enough to find it. Once you do, the rewards are great; in fact, they are life changing. Once you start changing your outlook, and instead of looking at what you can accomplish in your own strength; when you truly begin to have faith and belief in the works that God is doing in your life that you may or may not be able to see, you will be inviting the Holy Spirit to dwell inside you. He will begin to transform you into what God sees in you, what God wants for you, and what His plans are. I quadruple dog-dare you to try.

Go ahead, have a look.

I will wait.

I'm still waiting.

Go ahead.

Then I will get back to my mother visiting me that dreadful night.

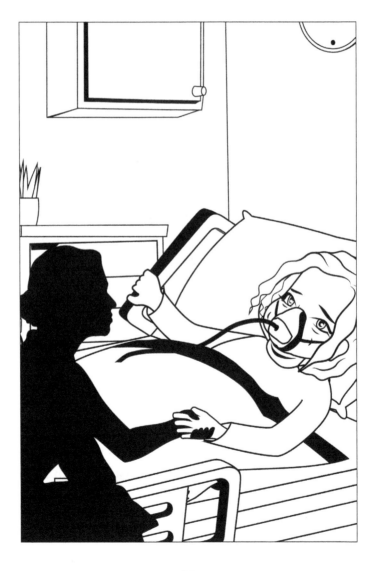

It was in the middle of the night when I was shaking, going deaf from the machines beeping and feeling so very alone when it happened. I felt a small, cold hand on my left hand. I looked over and saw a small silhouette of what appeared to be a very tiny, petite woman sitting next to my bed, holding my hand. It was as if she was telling me that I was going to be okay. Just over her shoulder, up against the wall was a much larger silhouette of a man. He was leaning up against the wall, just looking at me. He reminded me of my father-in-law. The small woman sitting next to me reminded me of my sweet mother.

They each had what appeared to be a shadow of a light around them. It was like they were slightly glowing a yellowish white color. They both looked happy and healthy but very concerned. Then the woman patted my hand one last time and smiled at me. The next thing I remembered; they both were gone. I have no idea how long that lasted; it could have been seconds, minutes, or even an hour. But at that moment, that precise moment, I knew I was going to be okay. I can't explain it; I just knew. That perfect storm of machines beeping, increasing anxiety and fear, culminated with my special visitors that night and the reassurance that I was in fact going to be okay. It was not my time.

I also knew I was extremely hypoxic. It would be easily explained that my brain lacked oxygen, and I was experiencing a hallucination. But I do not believe that. Now science and logic would tell you that I experienced a very emotional anxiety attack compounded by the lack of oxygen going to my brain, that I imagined the entire experience. They would think the lack of oxygen played tricks on my brain. Science would say I was hallucinating, but I know it was real. I know the feeling that suddenly came over me, the sensation I experienced, and the complete, utter peace that settled over me. For the first time, I knew what I needed to do.

I felt my dead mother's hand on my left hand. My heart rate started to slow down, and I felt my anxiety easing just from her hand holding mine. I don't care what science says, it was real. I know what

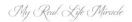

I experienced, and I believe to this day that it was real and what led to my life being saved. That was the starting point of my improvement. I didn't say a word of my experience to anyone, not even my husband. It wasn't until I had been home from the hospital for a few weeks when we approached the subject of how close they came to losing me.

My husband held my hand and then pulled me into a big bear hug and cried. He told me how scared he was, how scared everyone was, and that he didn't know what he would have done if they had lost me. I listened to his fears and reassured him that I wasn't going anywhere anytime soon; this was a once-in-a-lifetime kind of scare! I felt miserable that I had put my family through that misery; I ruined the holidays with my illness. My husband and son had to fend for themselves on Thanksgiving Day because they were quarantined. I didn't get to make Thanksgiving Dinner for my family, I didn't get to spend the holiday with my family, and to top it off, they spent the day wondering if I would make it through the day. Now I was ruining Christmas for my entire family. I was home but couldn't do anything but sit on my butt and suck down that oxygen.

My husband shared with me that he had never in his life prayed so hard as he did while I was in the hospital. He was terrified that I was going to die. The doctors kept calling him and telling him that I was minutes away from being put on the ventilator, and every call scared him ten times more. It was during one of these conversations that he shared with me that he was so scared that he started praying not only to God but started talking to both his dad and my mom, asking both to look after me. We realized that prayer happened on the same day I experienced by miracle, the day my mom and his dad visited me from heaven in my hospital room. It was at that moment I knew for sure I was going to be okay, the moment I knew that the only way out of this situation was to agree being put on the BIPAP.

It was that single, simple intervention that was going to change the course of my illness from serious to the road to recovery. The next morning, I still refused to sign that stupid DNR, but I did agree to going on BIPAP and being transferred to the ICU. If truth be told, I must have been a little sterner in my refusal of the ventilator and to sign the DNR because they stopped asking me every day. They were shocked that I had agreed to the BIPAP and didn't ask me a second time. I think they were scared I would change my mind because within minutes, I was on it.

As a nurse, I have witnessed many unexplainable events in my years. I have taken care of a lot of people who had died, some with family by their bedside and some alone with only me to hold their hand as they took their last breath. I have held too many hands to count and watched too many people take their last breath without any loved ones by their side. I have witnessed patients talking to people who were not there with them; I have witnessed people telling me they see a light and felt like they were supposed to go to the light. And as a nurse, I made any number of thousands of excuses for their behavior, the biggest being the elderly patient was sundowning; with younger people I just chalked it up to a reaction to the medications they were taking. I once had an elderly woman take my hand and tell me, "Sweetie, you have been so nice to me and my John just wanted you to know that he appreciated you being so kind to me, but it is soon time for me to go and join my love, John." I just patted her hand and told her to get some rest; no one was allowed to die on my watch. By morning, she was gone. Honestly, I have never forgotten that encounter. It has stuck with me all this time.

It is a well-known phenomenon that people will see and talk to dead people right before they are going to die. You hear these stores all the time, and I have witnessed several of them myself. Wasn't this happening to me? But somehow, I just knew I was going to be okay. I just knew it. I had such an overwhelmingly sense of peace about me at that one particular moment. My heart rate had slowed down and wasn't as erratic. My breathing slowed down. and I was no longer hyperventilating. And, while I didn't sleep, I was at ease. I put on a bedtime story narrated by Matthew McConaughey and easily slipped into a sense of complete calmness. Not sleep but calmness.

Here I was, isolated from everyone and anyone that I loved and that loved me. I had no one to talk to because I just couldn't breathe. I was all alone in this dark, lonely hospital room, and I had angelic visitors to reassure me and to give me the confidence to fight and survive. God wasn't done with me yet. I had work to do. This was not how my story was going to end. In that moment, I made a promise to do better, to *be* better. A promise I will keep the rest of my life.

Healing Miracles of the Bible

M iracles are mentioned throughout the Bible. We have all heard about them, haven't we? *This is another good time to put the book down, grab your coffee and do a little more self-reflection. Do you really believe in miracles? Have you ever experienced something yourself that you could not explain? Well, have you? Be honest.*

As a nurse, I have often seen people who were supposed to be dying, suddenly recover. Someone lived, who by all accounts should not be alive. I saw this many, many times in the emergency room. I saw someone live who had been shot at point blank range right into the heart. I know medicine tries to explain it. Surgeons brilliantly and skillfully went in and surgically removed the bullet, with no damage or very little damage done to the heart muscle. The excuse made was that he was young and healthy, or credit is given to a skillful surgeon and the patient getting to the emergency room very quickly. I get it.

But now I know—it was God. It was a miracle sent straight from above. Yes, the surgeon and medical personnel are very skilled and knowledgeable, but it was God who gave them the knowledge to do what they do. God set all the right things in motion; God put the right people in those circumstances to save that life. God guided those well-trained hands to tend to those wounds. Miracles are strange occurrences that happen in the world that have no natural explanation. I know that now just as sure as I am breathing on my own right now without that stupid oxygen tube in my nose.

Faith is key—you just have to believe. Have you figured out a theme?

Get ready, as my husband always says, "It's time for me to do some Bible surfing."

The greatest of *all* miracles is Jesus. We can't write about miracles without starting with this one. In John 14:11 (NIV), Jesus says to his disciples,

> *"Believe me that I am in the Father and the Father is in me, or at least believe on the evidence of miracles themselves."*

God used miracles to demonstrate his power over nature; God used miracles to reign over the nations and all people, to show victory over death, to heal the sick, to warn of judgment; to show superiority over false gods. He used miracles to provide for the needs of His people, to show love and compassion, and finally, to show His plan for salvation.

The miracle of healing the sick is discussed in the Bible in *three* different books, each describing one of *twenty-three* different instances of the sick being healed. I am starting with this example because while all are of equal importance, this book of course, is about the miracle of healing, so why not start there? Besides, I experienced a miracle of healing, so this particular type of miracle pulls at the heart strings. Wouldn't it for you?

The first example is in 2 Kings 5:10–14 (NIV),

> *"Elisha sent a messenger to say to him, go wash yourself seven times in the Jordan and your flesh will be restored and you will be cleansed."*

Let's back up just a little to the beginning of 2 Kings, chapter 5 (NIV), where we learn that Naaman, a great commander of the army of King Aram had leprosy. Naaman was sent by his master, King

Aram, to seek out Elisha so he could be cured of his leprosy. Elisha's instructions to the great commander were to go to the Jordan and cleanse himself in the river, a dirty river I might add, not once but seven times. Even though he went away angry, he did indeed take a dip in the Jordan seven times as instructed. His flesh was restored and clean just like it was when he was a little boy. Who would have ever thought bathing yourself in a dirty river seven times would heal someone of leprosy? But that is exactly what happened; Naaman was healed of his leprosy.

In 2 Kings, chapter 20, our second example, we find that Hezekiah fell ill and was going to die from this illness. But Hezekiah had been a faithful and loyal servant to the Lord God. Many prayers were prayed, and many tears shed in hopes of God healing him. Finally, he was instructed to go to the temple of the Lord on the third day, and the Lord would add fifteen years to his life. 2 Kings 20:7 (NIV) tells us:

> *"Then Isaiah said, Prepare a poultice of figs. They did so*
> *and applied it to the boil and he recovered."*

Hezekiah had been a loyal and trusted king of Jerusalem for twenty-nine years, and God healed him of his illness, sparing his life for fifteen more years.

Our third example of healing in the Bible is in Matthew 8:1–4 (NIV), where we see another man with leprosy:

> *"When he came down from the mountainside, large crowds*
> *followed him. A man with leprosy came and knelt before*
> *him and said Lord, if you are willing, you can make me*
> *clean. Jesus reached out his hand and touched the man. I*
> *am willing he said, Be clean! Immediately he was cured*
> *of his leprosy."*

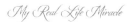

Jesus was known for healing many from all kinds of different ailments, but this example in Matthew 8 demonstrates that all you had to do was ask and believe. Jesus was not stingy on his miracles of healing. He wanted to heal people, even the common town folk. He just wanted to help people. After all, He is the only human being ever, who was perfect in all ways. He loved everyone, regardless of social class, income, race, sex, and especially if you weren't too perfect.

In Matthew 9:1–8 (NIV) Jesus healed a paralytic man:

> *Jesus stepped into a boat, crossed over and came to his own town. Some men brought to him a paralytic, lying on a mat. When Jesus saw their faith, he said to the paralytic, take heart, son, your sins are forgiven. At this time of the teachers of the law said to themselves, this fellow is blaspheming! Knowing their thoughts, Jesus said why do you entertain evil thoughts in your hearts? Which is easier: to say, your sins are forgiven or to say get up and walk? But so that you may know that the son of man has authority on earth to forgive sins, then he said to the paralytic, get up, take your mat and go home. And the man got up and went home. When the crowd saw this, they were filled with awe; and they praised God, who had given such authority to men.*

Let's look at the last example, recorded in Mark 8:22–26 (NIV). Here we find Jesus at it again, this time healing the blind:

> *They came to Bethsaida and some people brought a blind man and begged Jesus to touch him. He took the blind man by the hand and let him outside of the village. When he had spit on his eyes and put his hands on him, Jesus asked do you see anything? He looked up and said I see people, they look like trees walking around. Once more,*

Jesus put his hands on the man's eyes. Then his eyes were opened, his sight was restored, and he saw everything clearly. Jesus sent him home saying don't go into the village.

Finally, in John 3, a beggar was healed by Peter. This man was so grateful that he was seen walking the streets praising God instead of begging. I would say two miracles occurred here. The man was healed of his ailment, and he began to sing the praises of our Lord. Jesus didn't know these people, but He performed these miracles and healed total strangers. Let's face it, would you walk down the street and when you see someone sitting on a bench having an asthma attack, would you stop, put your hands on them, and tell them to breathe? No, you would not. Most people would just call 911, but there are those that would be too busy to stop and help at all.

How many times have you driven past an accident and kept on driving by? I think we might all be guilty of that. The way our society is today, you would be afraid of being shot. There are twenty-three instances of Jesus healing the sick described in the Bible. And I am sure there were many more. I could talk about these miracles all day! How many times have you said in your life when someone you knew or heard about on the news, who by all accounts should have died but didn't, "That was a miracle"? We use that term as if it an everyday occurrence, but have we ever really thought about those miracles? It's a miracle when that premature baby, who was born way too early and only weighed two pounds, lives a full life. Face it, miracles happen every day.

How about the miracles of Jesus raising the dead? Those people were cold- dead-dead-dead and dead. Let that sink in for a minute. He brought them back from the dead. There are *six* accounts in *four* different books. In 1 Kings 17:17–23(NIV), we find Elijah staying with the widow at Zarephath. Her son fell ill.

Sometime later the son of the women who owned the house became ill. He grew worse and worse, and finally stopped breathing. She said the Elijah, "What do you have against me, man of God? Did you come to remind me of my sins and kill my son?" Elijah replied, "Give me your son. He took him from her arms, carried him to the upper room where he was staying and laid him on his bed. Then he cried out to the Lord. "O Lord my God, have you brought tragedy also upon this widow I am staying with, by causing her son to die?" Then he stretched himself out on the boy three times and cried to the Lord, "O Lord my God, let this boy's life return to him!" The Lord heard Elijah's cry, and the boy's life returned to him, and he lived. Elijah picked up the child and carried him down from the room into the house. He gave him to his mother and said, "Look your son is alive!"

Elijah was a man of true faith and believed completely in God. He knew God would hear his cries and restore the boy's life, so it was done. In 2 Kings 4:19–37, we find Elisha who often visited a well-off woman; she always urged him to stay to eat. He came to Shunem, where this woman told her husband to make Elisha a room since she knew he was a man of God. Elisha promised this woman a son. In fact, he was very prescriptive on when this son would come. Just as Elisha predicted, the following year she had a son. In 2 Kings 4:19–37 (NIV), we read:

The child grew and one day he went out to his father, who was with the reapers, My head! My head! He said to his father. His father told the servant to take him to his mother. After the servant had lifted him up and carried him to his mother the boy sat on her lap until noon, then he died. She went up and laid him on the bed of the man of

*God, then shut the door and went out. She called her hus-
band and said "please send me one of the servants and a
donkey so I can go to the man of God quickly and return."
Why go to him today? He asked. It's not the new moon or
the sabbath. It's all right she said. She saddled the donkey
and said to her servant, "lead on don't slow down for me
unless I tell you." So she set out and came to the man
of God at Mount Carmel. When he saw her in the dis-
tance, the man of God said to his servant Gehazi "Look!
There's the Shunammite! Run to meet her and ask her
are you all right? Is your husband all right? Is your child
all right?" She replied everything was all right . . . When
Elisha reached the house, there was the boy lying dead on
his couch. He went in, shut the door on the two of them
and prayed to the Lord. He got on the bed and lay upon
the boy, mouth to mouth, eyes to eyes, hands to hands.
As he stretched himself out upon him, the boy's body grew
warm. Elisha turned away and walked back and forth
in the room and then got on the bed and stretched out
upon him once more. The boy sneezed seven times and
opened his eyes.*

In the book of Luke, we find the first of two examples of the dead
being raised. In Luke 7:11–17 (NIV), Jesus once again followed by
a large crowd and his disciples:

*As he approached the town gate, a dead person was being
carried out—the only son of his mother and she was a
widow. And a large crowd from the town was with her.
When the Lord saw her, his heart went out to her and he
said, "Don't cry." Then he went up and touched the coffin
and those carrying it stood still. He said, "young man, I*

*say to you, get up!" The dead man sat up and began to
talk, and Jesus gave him back to his mother.*

In John, chapter 11, Lazarus who was the brother to Mary, was
very sick. Lazarus was the brother to Mary. Remember Mary? She
was the one that poured perfume on Jesus's feet and wiped his feet
with her hair. John 11:4 (NIV)states:

> *When he heard of this, Jesus said "This sickness will not
> end in death. No, it is for God's glory so that God's son
> may be glorified through it."*

But when Jesus arrived, he found that Lazarus had already been
dead and in the tomb for four days. Jesus promised that Lazarus
would rise again. John 11:40–44 (NIV) states:

> *Then Jesus said, "Did I not tell you that if you believed,
> you would see the glory of God?" So they took away the
> stone. Then Jesus looked up and said, "Father, I thank you
> that you have heard me. I knew that you always hear me
> but I said this for the benefit of the people standing here,
> that they may believe that you sent me."*

> *When he had said this, Jesus called in a loud voice,
> "Lazarus come out!" The dead man came out, his hands
> and feet wrapped with strips of linen, and a cloth around
> his face. Jesus said to them, "take off the grave clothes and
> let him go."*

And it was so. Lazarus rose from the dead. And let's not forget the
greatest miracle of raising the dead, the resurrection of Christ. Have
you heard about this one? Jesus was brutally murdered on a cross and
rose three days later. In Luke 24: 6–7 (NIV), the angel said:

He is not here; he has risen! Remember how he told you, while he was still with you in Galilee: The son of man must be delivered into the hands of sinful men, be crucified and on the third day be raised again.

Three days after being crucified and placed in the tomb, Jesus rose again, just as the Father and Son had promised.

What kind of book would this be if we didn't mention the plagues noted in the Bible. After all, this is a book about my bout as a COVID long hauler, the latest world-famous plague to hit take the world by storm. Everyone has been touched by this pandemic.

In Exodus 7:20–21 (NIV) we find:

Moses and Aaron did just as the Lord had commanded. He raised his staff in the presence of Pharaoh and his offi-cials and struck the water of the Nile, and all the water was changed into blood. The fish in the Nile died, and the river smelled so bad that the Egyptians could not drink its water, blood was everywhere in Egypt.

Take a moment an meditate about these miracles I have described and maybe even dust off that old Bible and read them for yourself. Think about where our world is right now and the parables between our current situation in the United States as well as throughout the entire world. How much of what is happening or has happened in recent years reminds you of God's demonstration of power of the nations and people? These miracles tell us one thing for sure. Every person in the Bible that experienced a miracle believed, had faith and just knew beyond a shadow of doubt what they believed was the absolute truth.

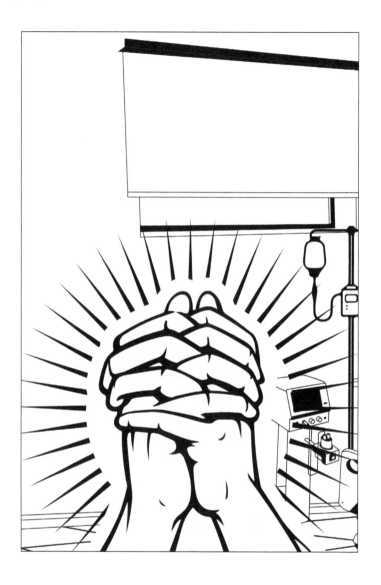

Nurses are the Heartbeat of the Medical Field

This is my soapbox alert and my plug for nurses near and far! Let's clear up any misconceptions, shall we? The nursing profession is misunderstood and lacks the respect they most certainly deserve. Nurses are the backbone of the healthcare field and the heartbeat of the healthcare industry. Nursing is the largest profession in the healthcare industry consisting of roughly three million strong but also the largest workforce inside an industry that was hit hard by a pandemic that was gripping the world. When COVID hit, it took not only the healthcare industry by storm, but also negatively impacted the nursing profession. Nurses spend the most time with the patients in any scenario, but when COVID struck, the nurses now faced a dilemma; too many patients were flooding the emergency rooms, being admitted, and they suddenly found themselves carrying an extremely high load of patients to care for. Combine that with fear of taking the virus home to loved ones, and nurses were left with the perfect storm of healthcare. Nurses were told to limit the time spent in the room with COVID patients; not to linger; do your tasks and get out. I can remember spending time in rooms with my patients, completing my assessments or giving medications and chit chatting with them or conversing over what they were watching. COVID stopped the small talk.

They had too many patients to care for, who were coming in at an alarming rate. The nurse-to-patient ratio was too high. There just were not enough nurses to care for all these sick people who were flooding the emergency rooms. COVID units were created to contain the virus, and nurses were pulled or hired to work these units. We were learning along the way. It was not a great environment for anyone involved—and a very precarious situation for all involved. Honestly, the medical field was learning on the fly. Patients were being admitted so fast that it was putting an unfamiliar burden on the healthcare industry. Nurses were struggling with too many extremely sick patients to care for and not really having a full understanding of this virus. Medical surgical nurses were now being expected to be critical care nurses caring for patients on monitors. Something that was definitely a change from their normal practice.

I struggled when it was time to pull outpatient nurses to the inpatient units to care for these patients. Although I completely understood the rationale behind the decision, I had a tough time wrapping my head around what we were asking nurses to do. Some of the nurses were single parents who had to send their babies to stay with family so they would not infect them. Others with high-risk family members had to live in a hotel to avoid making them sick. I just could not get past that. The sacrifice we were asking them to make weighed heavily on my heart and was just unfathomable. Nurses who were close to retirement age; had not worked on an inpatient unit for over twenty years, found themselves back to shift work on an inpatient unit. Unimaginable.

Come on now, you expected a plug for nurses. I am not going to disappoint. Nurses work hard, often without a break in a twelve-hour shift. The bladder inside a nurse is as strong as a steel drum. I can remember numerous times never going to the bathroom at all during a busy shift, not one time and never even getting a chance to grab a drink of water. When I was a floor nurse, I often had too many patients to care for at once by myself. The nurse-to-patient ratio has always been high.

In the emergency room, I can remember coming in one Saturday evening for the start of my 1900 shift to see a tour bus parked outside the emergency room doors, eight ambulances in the ambulance bay, and every bed filled with patients, while the waiting room was standing room only. In the dressing room (because this was before the day when you were allowed to wear your scrubs home—*gross*), I was wondering where the other night-shift nurses were. I changed into my scrubs and walked into the emergency room. It was me and one other nurse for the night shift. We relieved eight day-shift nurses. Diane and I looked at each other and said, "I have the even numbered beds, you got the odd numbered, and we will rotate traumas." And that is how we started our shift. Before we knew it, a nurse came in at 2300. That was a relief. And about 0300, it finally slowed down, and we were finally able to come up for air. My point is nurses work like this all the time. Nurses get sick, have kids that get sick, and are just downright exhausted. They go an entire shift without a bio-break. They go an entire shift without eating or drinking. Sometimes they go an entire shift without even noticing what the weather is like outside or what time it is. Sometimes they go an entire shift without carrying on a conversation with another staff member.

There has been a severe nursing shortage for years, for as long as I can remember. If I think back to the beginning of my nursing career, we have always had a severe nursing shortage, so short that the nurse-to-patient ratio has always been at an unsafe level. Yes, hospitals do their best to recruit the best candidates, train them well, and attempt to retain good nurses. The problem is nurses get burned out really fast. No, patients don't notice the shortage because we do an excellent job caring for our patients. We hide the misery and exhaustion from showing on our faces. We smile, we laugh, we care, and yes, we cry. We hold hands when hands need to be held. We give medications when they are due. We answer all the questions from loved ones. We let family members yell and vent at us. We educate patients and families. Nursing is a caring profession. And so, we care for the patient and the family. It takes a special kind of person to become a nurse. Caring is a spiritual gift; a gift that requires a lot of sacrifices, a lot of compassion and empathy.

When COVID hit the United States and the World, it not only took the population by surprise, but the healthcare professionals as well. The virus was spreading at a rapid rate. People were dying. Thousands of people were critically ill, and emergency rooms were being overrun. The news painted a very desolate picture. Images of healthcare providers looking distraught, overwhelmed, and utterly exhausted filled every news channel and newspaper. Nurses, just like the rest of the population, were afraid. The lack of knowledge regarding this virus fed the fear.

Nurses were forced to live apart from their families in fear of bringing the virus home to loved ones. Isolation was a real threat to the healthcare industry and society. Isolation caused increased fear. Increased fear caused more isolation. It was a never-ending vicious cycle. Nurses are taught in school how important it is to care for the whole patient, and that includes involving the family in the care and in the decision-making process. And here we were, isolating patients from their loved ones during a time when they truly needed to be together, whether it was to hold a hand and will them to fight or kiss them and say goodbye.

When patients are on a ventilator, it is crucial for families to sit at the bedside, hold the hands of the loved one, and talk to them. It is key for them to be present, and research shows it has a positive impact on recovery. Including the family members during bedside rounds helps promote family involvement in decisions for care, and the use of FaceTime just can't replace being present in the moment. We are just now realizing the impact of the isolation of both the nurses and the patients during the pandemic. The mind, spirit and body took a serious blow from the isolation. I know all to well, the impact it has had on this nurse turned patient. My experience has forced me to have a whole new outlook on the nurse-patient relationship and I have noticed a change in the nurse in me as a result.

Hospitals were converting wards to COVID wards. Normal hospital rooms were turned into private rooms with monitors installed. Regular rooms converted into monitored, negative-pressure rooms. Staff were being pulled from everywhere to work these newly formed units. Staff were pulled from outpatient settings, from the operating room, or from other wards. Nurses were given a quick down-and-dirty orientation to the new ward and were taught what the medical profession knew up to that point about COVID: how to treat it, how to care for these patients, and most importantly, how to prevent the spread. Some of these nurses had not worked an inpatient unit for decades; some never had. And here we were, plucking them out of their environment, the one they were probably subject matter experts on and plopping them right into an uncomfortable and unknown situation, caring for patients who were very critically ill. There were even nurses coming out of retirement to help care for these patients.

This is what I struggled with the most in my role in nursing leadership. I kept imagining what I would feel like if that were me. I know I would not have liked it. I would have felt set up to fail. And, I know I would not have been happy about it. But that is exactly what we did. Honestly, we didn't have a choice. But our nurses stepped up to plate and hit a homerun. They did what they always do and rose to the occasion. But at what cost to their mental health and wellbeing? I'm afraid it will be years before we truly understand the impact.

The patients were being admitted at a precipitous rate, and the healthcare field had to think on their feet how to best care for these patients. I had never seen anything like this in my entire career. This was the most doable and best that could be done quickly. We did not have time to put nurses through a six-week orientation process. Nurses who had not worked in years were being hired, put through an expeditious orientation process and then put on these wards to care for very sick patients. Sometimes I thought we were hiring anyone with a license. As long as they could work, they were hired. Heck, as long as they had a heartbeat and were willing, we were putting them to work. We did the best we could, given the circumstances. Truthfully, , as a nurse who experienced this type of nursing as a patient, I have to say, we must do better. I was isolated from my family. I felt isolated from the staff. I was isolated from the outside world. I felt as if life was continuing on around me, and I was stuck in some sort of *Groundhog Day* nightmare. My hospital door was kept closed at all times. The medical professionals only came in the room when needed and only for as long as it took to complete their tasks. I could not even carry on a conversation with them. Some did linger a few extra minutes but most, especially during that first few days or weeks, came in and left just as fast. I was contagious after all.

Once transferred to the ICU and then the step-down unit, my experience was a little different. The door to my room was still kept closed, but the staff seemed to spend a little more time in my room than they did on the COVID unit. Maybe I wasn't considered contagious anymore. Just imagine being kept shut up in a room with only the TV to keep you company. People were coming in and out for just a few minutes at a time, dressed in banana suits. All you could truly see was their eyes. There was no real human contact the entire time you are in the hospital, and most patients hospitalized with COVID during the initial phase of this virus spent weeks to months in the hospital. Just imagine it. Just imagine the ongoing consequences of that isolation.

I pray that whoever is reading this will never experience anything like that. I watched the Hallmark Christmas shows over and over. I watched Fox News Channel over and over. I listened to my Bible app over and over. I know during the time where I was extremely hypoxic, that I probably talked to myself. I was miserable. I was lonely. I was craving human contact.

The lack of empathy from the healthcare personnel was astounding. I was amazed at how little empathy I felt from the majority of the staff. Some were really good, and you could just feel the care and concern they had for me but others, not so much. I am not sure if it came from fear of the virus, lack of knowledge, fear of the unknown, or exhaustion on their part. Or all the above. I don't always tell people that I am a nurse but because this was COVID and everyone wanted to explore where the source of my particular infection came from, I let the cat out of the bag and just had to tell them that I was a nurse. They put it together and determined one plus one truly does equal two—I got it from work.

So, it is not like the staff were not all aware that I was a nurse, they knew. Or at least if they read my chart, they knew. But still I felt like I was all alone on this unit. I had to be my own advocate. The nurses were not going to be patient advocates in this situation. I am sure everyone expected me to die. No one thought I would ever go home. In fact, I remember the night I was being discharged, one of the nurses who took care of me on nightshift when I was first admitted and probably one of the only ones to show empathy came into my room to tell me that if I didn't go home, she was going to be my nurse that night. When I was being wheeled out in the wheelchair, she stopped me, gave me a hug, and told me she had been so scared for me. She thought for sure I was dying. She was very happy I was going home. I don't remember her name, but I remember her face, and I always will. I hope one day I see her again to tell her thank you for caring for me. So, whoever you are I say thank you from the bottom of my heart. While I don't remember your name, I remember you and I am truly grateful for you and the care you gave me.

I like to think I am a very strong person, emotionally, physically, and mentally. This experience has definitely taken a toll on me, and now I have my doubts on just how strong I really am. I am not as strong as I once was. I am filled with fear. I am terrified of getting COVID again. I am petrified of being around anyone with COVID.

When my husband got COVID for a second time this past summer, I was paralyzed with fear. We stayed in separate rooms for the entire quarantined period, but I was still unable to shake that feeling of doom. I am fearful when someone comes into my office. Even though we are still wearing surgical masks at work, I am still scared of being in close contact with anyone. I am certainly not comfortable getting on an elevator with a bunch of other people.

I have nightmares of being trapped in a box or a room or even a trunk of a car and not being able to escape. I feel like I am suffocating. I hate that. I have woken up in a sweat, looking around the room and immediately reaching out to touch my husband or even one of my dogs just so that I know I am not back in the hospital, and I am okay. I have disturbed my husband and my poor Harley girl a few times when I screamed in my sleep.

Another problem healthcare workers faced was the lack of personal protective equipment (PPE) and cleaning supplies due to the global supply-chain shortages. Suddenly it was acceptable to reuse masks and gowns. Proper PPE was vital to the healthcare staff to prevent the spread of the virus and to keep them from getting sick too. Reusing PPE was mind-blowing to me. Surgical masks and N95s were not meant to be worn for twelve-hour shifts. Wear it; then throw it away. Not wear it, leave it on the entire shift, and then take it off and put it in a paper lunch bag and keep it in your locker when you don the mask you went into work with. If you could not pass the N95 fit test, you were given a PAPR, a powered air purifying respirator to wear. This looks like a Martian suit from old movies. Healthcare workers who can't pass the fit test to wear N95 are issued these types of personal protection. There was no way that anyone who could physically work, would not be working.

What in the world was going on? We had all lost our minds. I remember how I felt and what went through my mind when it was announced that it was now okay to reuse our PPEs due to the severe shortage of supplies. Ridiculous. Being a nurse was different than it was thirty years ago. We were wearing our surgical masks every day until it was soiled, then we were allowed to be issued another one. I had never seen anything like this before.

I read something recently that stated over 200,000 healthcare workers left the workforce in 2021 alone. The pandemic has caused many to rethink careers and to reprioritize goals. Physician, nurses, nurse practitioners, and other healthcare workers were fleeing the profession to pursue owning businesses, consulting, or other careers completely. Others were not leaving the profession but were leaving direct patient care. A lot of people lost loved ones, colleagues, and friends, causing a different outlook on their professional life and personal lives. I personally know several that retired. The healthcare industry was already at a critical staffing level, especially for nurses, and the pandemic only shattered an already-stressed profession.

The nurses on the COVID ward where I was admitted were no different. They were tired, overworked, and scared. They had seen too much death. I remember one day when I was in the ICU, I could see through the window looking into the rest of the ICU a patient across the nursing station from me, who must not have been doing well. He or she coded and did not survive. I did not see a nurse for hours. Let me repeat that, I did *not* see a nurse for *hours*. No one came in my room to check on me, not even when I pressed the call bell. It was like they all went home and left the patients all alone. I could not hear anyone talking. I could not hear anyone going in or out of rooms. I heard lots of beeping from machines in other rooms, including mine, yet I did not see a nurse for hours

Finally, a very young nurse came into my room and introduced himself as taking over my care for the remainder of the dayshift. I had never seen this guy before, and quite honestly, he didn't look old enough to shave or drive; yet here he was, taking care of me. I have been in situations where we lost patients before. We did do debriefs, but we never abandoned our patients in the middle of the shift. The only thing that I can surmise is that it must have been one of them in that room across from me, and the loss was understandably devastating to all in that unit. The young nurse, who came in to care for me, had been pulled to that unit. He was very sweet and attended to my needs, but the entire situation had piqued my curiosity and I have never forgotten it.

Nursing, by trade, is a compassionate profession. We have empathy for the patients entrusted to us. We care for the patient and the family simultaneously spending more time with our patients than any other healthcare worker. We bathe our patients, get them up out of bed and back to bed, assist them to the bathroom, and we feed them; not to mention administering any number of other IVs, medications, or other treatments that keep us in the patients' rooms. Nurses have such a positive impact on the outcomes of our patients. Even back in the days of Florence Nightingale, credited with starting the profession, nurses decreased the death toll at the hospital where she worked. This was long before nursing was considered a profession.

One thing we have been taught as nurses is how important it is to involve the family in the treatment of their loved ones and how important it is to have family at the bedside with anyone who is hospitalized and especially those in critical condition. Outcomes can be influenced by having a loved one sit and talk with the patient. Even patients on ventilators can respond to hearing a loved one's voice or feeling the touch of their hand. And here we were, isolating patients from their loved ones. I can't tell you the impact that had on me. I didn't realize it at the time, but looking back and remembering my experience has proven to me the significance of seeing my family. I did not see my husband or my children the entire time I was hospitalized, and I don't care what the subject matter experts tell you. FaceTime and Zoom calls cannot replace having someone who loves me at the bedside talking to me and holding my hand.

The isolation that I experienced has had an adverse effect on me. I have nightmares. I dream that I am locked in a room or a box by myself and I can't escape. I can hear voices, but I can't escape. This virus has caused so many damaging consequences on my life. I suffer from PTSD. Not only do I have nightmares, but I am terrified of being alone. There has been two times since coming home that my husband has had to go out of town, and I was terrified to be alone. Granted, I am never truly alone. I have four dogs at my house but not having another human there with me was distressing.

We were trying to keep our patients safe, trying to protect others from getting COVID, and trying to protect the healthcare workers; but I do not think we thought about the long-term consequences of the isolation of patients with COVID, not just in the hospital setting but being forced to quarantine in our homes. Not seeing your family. Not being able to attend family gatherings, weddings, birthday celebrations and yes, even funerals was detrimental to the mental wellbeing of our very population. The lockdown affected everyone much the same way, our children as well as the adults. Children need socialization to grow and learn how to interact with others and yet, we isolated them as well.

The increase in mental illness, depression, and suicides because of the isolation have contributed to the ever-increasing burden on the healthcare system. I think the consequences of such widespread isolation has yet to be determined. Patients hospitalized in the ICUs are at higher risk for Post Intensive Care Syndrome (PICS) which simply means there are several health problems that remain after a critical illness. PICS also puts one at risk for developing depression and PTSD. Isolation can also result in depression and PTSD. I have never suffered from depression or mental illness before, but now I suffer from nightmares and overwhelming sense of fear. I can't stress this enough. I am afraid of being alone. I am afraid of getting COVID again, in fact, that alone can cause me to have a full-blown panic attack, and I am afraid of being locked in somewhere and not being able to escape. I hate how this fear has paralyzed me. I regularly feel like I am stuck in a new prison.

I often wonder how many nurses suffer from depression and PTSD from working during the pandemic caring for these patients, watching one after another die. How many of them have nightmares? Have healthcare systems started offering mental health counseling for them? Is this part of the reason for the mass exodus from the healthcare profession? Has anyone thought of them? Does anyone care about the impact this pandemic has had on everyone in this world? Did we give evil doers carte blanche to destroy our lives? Or did we set the stage for more people to experience miracles?

Going Home!

Saturday came, and a new physician came to see me. He was not very sympathetic to my desire to go home. No amount of charm, charisma or convincing was going to win this guy over. He was immune to it all. I resigned myself to my current situation, and I informed my husband that I wouldn't be home until Monday or Tuesday at the earliest. We both had adjusted to that fact; I felt defeated in my quest to be home over the weekend and before my birthday and especially before my son made the trek across the country.

It was very depressing thinking that I would not get the chance to see my son off and to tell him how proud I was that he was following his dreams. He was starting a new chapter of his life and I was not home to see it. Then about 4 p.m., I got a call from an oxygen company verifying my home address. They were going to deliver a portable oxygen tank to me at the hospital after they delivered oxygen equipment to my house. The nurse came in as I was hanging up and told me she just saw discharge orders on me!

I was going home, escaping my prison! I was finally going home after what seemed like a lifetime. I was elated and scared, but the happiness won out! I didn't care what was to come; I was going home.

I called my husband and gave him the good news! I was coming home! I was on six liters of oxygen and still very ill, but I was going home! After discovering the hospital had lost my pants during the many transfers I had, and after sending my husband back home to get a pair of sweats for me to put on, I was finally in a wheelchair, headed

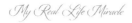

down the hall toward the elevator. I had tears streaming down my face, and some of the nurses stopped me in the hall and told me how glad they were I was going home. A few, who were there the night I was admitted, had tears in their eyes too. They were so happy things didn't end the way everyone expected them to. Some even stated they never thought I would make it home, but they were so happy I had a *God-sized miracle*.

I got in the elevator still crying and then, once on the ground floor, I could see my husband standing next to my car eagerly waiting on me. At that moment, I wanted to get out of that wheelchair and run into his waiting arms. I wanted to feel his strength as if it was all I needed to give me strength. The nurse wheeled me outside, and my husband was so excited to see me that he started fist pumping the air. They helped me in the car, got all my stuff loaded in the trunk and the oxygen bottle situated in the car, and I was on my way home!

Let the work begin! I had a long haul ahead of me, but no one, not even me, could have expected exactly how long.

My husband and son had cleared the driveway so my car could be pulled all the way up as close to the house as possible, and I wouldn't have to walk far. My husband had picked me up in my car because there was no way I could get up in his big ole' Ram Truck! My house is a rancher, so the only step I had to worry about was the one step up into the front door. I was never so glad not to have steps in my house. My husband pulled my brand spanking new walker (Yippee!) out of the trunk, got my oxygen bottle situated and helped me out of the car. It was time to take what seemed like the longest walk of my life! I had not taken more than two steps at a time since walking into the emergency room a few weeks prior.

I used the walker, and my husband pushed the oxygen tank behind me. My son had made sure my fur babies were outside so I could get to the bedroom without them jumping on me. He met me at the door, and between he and my husband, they got me into the house. My son helped me with the walker because I was so weak, I could not even push it. They got me into the house and into the bedroom. It was not pretty.

I was so thankful it was dark outside by the time I got home so no one could see how pitiful I looked. Normally, when I step outside of my house, my hair and makeup is done to perfection, and I was definitely not looking like my normal self. I was one *hot mess!* When I finally got to the bedroom and was sitting on the bed, I could see myself in the mirror and was shocked. I didn't even recognize myself. I was pale, frail, and looking old.

One by one, my fur babies came in to see me. I got love, kisses, and tail wags from Cassie, my Border Collie; Oreo and Merlot, my two litter-mate Pit Bull mixes; and Harley, my Pit Bull mix who was the newest member of the family. My son had cooked dinner, and the three of us sat on the bed and ate dinner together. That was the best pizza I had ever had in my life. That night, I had to sleep sitting up on five or six pillows. My husband became my nurse and took care of me. He cooked, cleaned, and did the laundry. He brought me meals in the bedroom. He had to dress me and help me to do everything little thing. I coughed all night, but my husband had things under control. He turned out to be such a great nurse!

Every time I got up, my oxygen sats dropped back into the eighties, and I would start coughing. The cough was ferocious and sometimes violent. He rubbed my back and talked to me until the coughing would subside and my sats came back up. He helped me prone every day. He took my vital signs twice every day. He literally was my lifeline. He showered me, washed my hair, and prepped my toothbrush for me. He even brought my makeup to me so I could do my face when I was feeling up to it. He helped me blow dry my hair and held my hand when I needed help calming my cough or breathing.

It gave a new meaning to the vows we took over thirty-five years ago—to have and to hold in sickness and in health. It was quite the eye opener; never in a million years did we expect COVID to affect us this way. When I came home, we never imagined exactly how hard things would be. We especially did not expect me to be home on six liters of oxygen. I do not know what we would have done if we both had not had a medical background. I probably would have gone to a long-term rehab facility instead of coming home. The normal lay person could not have done what we had to do, especially since I was discharged with no orders to follow except "follow up with your PCP." Unbelievable.

I am not even sure how we managed it all. It was so bad, and I was so weak, that I could not even cry. Crying made me gasp for breath, and it took too long to recover. The coughing hurt. Breathing hurt. My husband had to help me move around in the bed. I know I have said it before, but I am going to say it again, I was a *hot mess*. But it felt so good to be home. I had missed my own bed. I had missed my husband and my son and my dogs—all four of those loud mouths.

I finally got to see my youngest son the weekend after I came home. He surprised me for my birthday. He came with my daughter-in-law and grandson. I was so very surprised and so very happy. It felt so good to see my family, to get and give hugs and just see their smiling faces. It was the best feeling to see the worry wash away from their faces. I can't imagine what they had been going through. Our daughter lives in Texas with her husband, and she couldn't make the trip, but I heard it in her voice and saw it in her face when we zoomed. It was so clear on all their faces how scared they had been. I hate that I put them through that.

Reflections from David

Home, home at last. We had been hoping for a few days that Lisa would be well enough to come home soon. We knew that it wasn't going to be easy and that she was going to have a long road ahead of her, but I just knew that if I could get her home, I could give her the care that she really needed right now to recover. On Saturday, she said that if everything was stable and she was able to do a six-minute walk test, then they would discharge her to home. I was ecstatic at the thought of that happening. I dropped to my knees and thanked God for this chance and for making Lisa well enough to come home. I prayed and thanked Him for at least an hour. It was probably the longest I have ever prayed continuously in my entire life.

Lisa was coming home on six liters of oxygen, weak and needing help with everything she did. I was ready. I always wondered why I had spent so many years in the medical field. When I enlisted in the Navy many years ago, I had been a concrete finisher while in high school. After graduation and one year of college I decided to join the Navy. I wanted to be a Seabee (Navy construction worker), but there was a two-year wait.

I didn't want to wait, so the recruiter suggested that I become a Navy Hospital Corpsman. I had no idea what that was, but he explained it to me, so I decided to go for it. Little did I know that decision was all part of God's plan. This moment was the answer and reason as to why I became a corpsman. I had taken care of thousands

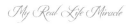

of sick and injured people during my career. Every experience was preparing me for the most important patient of my life, my wife.

I thanked God over and over for this chance to see my beautiful wife again and hold her in my arms. The oxygen company came to the house and set up the home oxygen. Shortly thereafter, I headed to the hospital to bring home the love of my life. We had shared everything in our lives to this point, so how bad could this be?

I arrived at the front door of the main hospital and parked as close as I could to the front door. It was dark outside and a little chilly. A nurse brought Lisa down to the parking lot in a wheelchair, and as she stood up, I could see that she was very weak. I helped her and the oxygen into the car. As we drove away, I just kept looking at the road, then at Lisa, then the road and back at Lisa. I just couldn't believe she was here, in the car and going home with me. I had a walker in the car because when we arrived at home, she needed to walk from the car into the front door and to our bedroom. Once there, we got her settled, and I gave her a huge hug and didn't want to let her go.

Over the next few days, I kept thanking God in my prayers and just watching her, so thankful that we had been given a second chance. The first couple of nights, I didn't sleep very well. I just kept waking up to make sure that she was still breathing. Lisa is a very strong woman, but she needed help with just about everything. I even learned how to shave her legs, and I got pretty good at it!

During the next few weeks, we were able to ween her from six liters of oxygen to not needing it at all. This wasn't as easy as it sounds. She would become very anxious and scared if I told her that we were going to turn her oxygen down today. So, I began doing it without telling her and when I did this, she did not become anxious. Little by little, she became more comfortable. She also was able to take short walks around the house (our house is only 1,700 square feet), though every time she was up on her feet for more than a minute, her heart rate would jump to the 130s or 140s. She would describe it as the feeling that she was running a marathon. That happened even when she took a shower and has continued to this day.

Skin breakdown was another thing that we were able to head off when getting her home. Prior to Lisa's illness, she was healthy, and her skin was always soft. It is ridiculous how fast someone's skin breaks down when they are sick and just lying in bed day in and day out. But we made sure that we moisturized her skin often throughout each day. If she had spent any more time in the hospital, her skin breakdown would have been much more difficult to manage. You see, because the nursing staff was so short-staffed and overworked, many of the seriously ill COVID-19 patients just laid in bed, unable to move themselves due to weakness or being unable to breathe. The simplest tasks were too difficult to perform. Laying in one position for too long caused pressure sores and skin breakdown.

The final thing that scared me to death upon her return home was leaving her alone at home while I returned to work. I was extremely scared to leave her. What if she had difficulty breathing, what if she fell, and what if she just wasn't strong enough to be on her own? We left all our concerns in God's hands. We just had to trust what He had in store.

Recovery

I had my first follow-up appointment via the phone with my primary care doctor. He was in shock that I had been discharged on six liters of oxygen and wanted me off the oxygen as quickly as possible. He did not truly understand exactly how sick I was. My husband started slowly turning it down every few days and turned it back up when necessary. I had been discharged with very few instructions. I had no instructions how to wean the oxygen or even when to start doing it. Who does that? Who discharges a patient who had been critically ill without any discharge instructions? That is just unimaginable.

After a week or so, my husband started helping me out to the living room so I could spend time with my son before he drove across the country to start his new life. I was only able to sit out there for an hour or two at first. After a few more weeks, my oxygen level was down to two liters! I was still coughing violently and still getting extremely short of breath when I was up on my feet, but I was holding steady at two liters.

After the first of the year, I was able to shower on my own, wearing my oxygen. My sats still dropped, but I began noticing my heart rate increasing dangerously high. It came back down to normal once I sat down. I was sent to Cardiology and Pulmonology. Both providers were shocked to see me. The cardiologist made the comment that I am the sickest person he had ever seen, and after reading my notes, he expected to see an old, frail-looking train wreck sitting in the exam room. Even though I felt like a frail, old train wreck, I must not have looked as bad as I thought I did! What a relief! My blood pressure was extremely high so, of course, here come the antihypertensive medications.

The pulmonologist expected to see a much sicker-looking woman in the exam room as well. She was surprised after seeing my hospital notes and scans that I was not worse off than I was. The pulmonologist informed me that I should continue to wean off the oxygen, and when I was able to come off completely, I could return to work full time in person. That was a surprise to us because I still had difficulty breathing, my heart rate was out of control, and my blood pressure was not controlled. I don't think she grasped fully how much walking I had to do at work or how big the facility was, where I worked.

The cardiologist determined I was able to return to work two days in person and three days teleworking a few months later, but going full time in person was out of the question. Remember the heart-rate issue? My heart rate was dangerously high after being upright only a few minutes. I was diagnosed with Postural Orthostatic Tachycardia (POTs) which is a condition that affects blood flow, and it is a syndrome of the Autonomic Nervous System. This system automatically controls and regulates vital body functions and activates the flight-or-fight response. It means my body cannot balance the way the vessels squeeze and pump blood throughout the body. When I stand and/or walk, my heart rate shoots up in the 100s. I get lightheaded, and the only thing that helps is to sit. In a nutshell, my regulator has taken a permanent vacation.

After a while, I began to realize that many of the symptoms I was experiencing were part of the syndrome now known as Long COVID or COVID long haulers. I was extremely fatigued, suffered from insomnia, and had headaches and nausea daily. I had extreme weakness and pain in my legs with muscle atrophy of my hamstrings and quadriceps. I had nightmares when I did actually fall asleep. I suffer from ongoing shortness of breath, post-exertional malaise, PTSD, severe brain fog, chronic cough, and rapid heart rate upon standing.

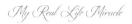

I have also been diagnosed with sleep apnea, tinnitus, and hearing loss due to COVID. In fact, there are several studies out there that can link the COVID virus to all the ailments I now have. There are also studies out there that suggest Long COVID mimics chronic fatigue syndrome.

Fifteen months from the start of this dreadful ordeal, I began pulmonary rehabilitation, twice a week for six weeks. During the intake session, the respiratory therapist was so positive and encouraging, telling me that they have had so many COVID patients, more than the normal patients you would see in Pulmonary Rehab. You know, the elderly with lung diseases, such as COPD. So, I was encouraged to start. You are going to feel so much better, just wait and see, he said. I had my doubts, but I was optimistic for the first time since this had begun. I was the only one not presently on oxygen, and I was the youngest. I was the only patient who was a COVID long hauler. No one else was recovering from COVID.

What I learned in the first two weeks was that patients being discharged from the hospital who had a rough time of it, on the ventilator or being discharged on oxygen are being sent right to Pulmonary Rehab very soon after hospitalization. Here I was, fifteen months since my diagnosis. I couldn't help but wonder, was it too little too late? In every session I did the same exercises, and it never got any easier, but I had made the decision before I started that I was going to give it everything I had. My quads and hamstrings screamed at me while I was on the treadmill; I had shortness of breath, but I told myself to "suck it up buttercup." The respiratory therapist told me over and over again that I looked stronger, but honestly, he had no clue what my body was going through. I just smiled and thanked him for the vote of confidence. Then I died once I got back into the car after each and every session.

They did not understand what the long hauler was going through, such as the extreme fatigue each session brought, the headache that came with each session as soon as I was done, and the exhaustion that made you want to crawl into bed and stay for days, but I couldn't do that. That meant I would be giving up, and I just couldn't do that, and I never would. I would push on even if I honestly didn't believe I would see much improvement. I couldn't help but wonder if this was too late, if the damage was already done. Time would tell. I was not being pessimistic; I was being realistic. I did not want to get my hopes up only to have them come crashing down with disappointment. I did it! I graduated Pulmonary Rehab, without ever missing a session everyone else missed several sessions. They were happy to see me finish and were thrilled I had "done so well."

Meanwhile, I wondered what was next. I didn't feel any improvement. I still couldn't breathe, my heart rate still skyrockets, and my legs were still so weak and hurt terribly. I didn't feel like I made any improvement at all. The nurse in me understands this is all new, but the patient in me is frustrated, and every shoulder shrug or scratch of the head frustrates me even more. It truly is discouraging when I have made it a point to educate myself on what COVID has done to me and continues to do and that my knowledge is greater than those who are charged with medically caring for me.

I am most likely facing retirement disability. And do you know what? I am ready for it. In fact, I am better than okay with it. I know that is the next chapter in our life together. My husband and I have come to accept it as the necessary next step in my road back to health.

God has a plan for me. He is the God of miracles and the God of Ephesians 3:20. He is the God of the impossible. Everyone thought it was impossible for me to get to this point. Let's face it, all the physicians who saw me did not think I had a snowball's chance to come home. Yet, here I am. Not only home, but I am functioning. Maybe not at the level I was before COVID, but I am here. I am breathing on my own. I am walking, perhaps like an old lady, but walking just the same.

Reflections from David

Wow, what can I say? This COVID has literally turned our lives upside down. My wife is the strongest person that I know. She has endured a lot, giving birth and raising three kids, twelve-hour night shifts in a busy emergency room, and taking care of my house and kids while I was deployed while in the service, but her past COVID illness and post COVID long hauler's ordeal has really been a challenge. Early on when she first came home, I thought that it would be a couple of weeks of recovery, and little by little, things would get back to normal. I don't think either of us imagined that two years later, she would still be dealing with this. Don't get me wrong, I am extremely grateful that we have this time together. But I worry about her mental health more than the physical.

She has many ailments associated with this long COVID, the worst of which is the extreme fatigue and increased heart rate she experiences with just taking thirty steps or being up on her feet for longer than a minute or two. The depression is what I worry about. To combat that, we have become extremely active at our church; teaching, mentoring, and organizing activities. We have even managed to take our camper out occasionally but, the walking, crossfitting, and hiking has been absent. Lisa continues to be a very motivated, determined person and passionate about life, but as two years leads to three and three to four years, what kind of toll is this taking on her emotionally? Our house is not very big, but it is comfortable. We have lived in this one-story rancher for thirty-two years, and though she often wishes for a larger home, it is hard not to wonder if this small house was part of God's plan.

For the most part, I do most of the cleaning and yard work. She continues to do the laundry, but I have to carry the clothes basket out to the laundry room each time. We love to cook together, listening to music while sipping a glass of wine. However, long COVID has even squashed that. Now we do still cook together, but she must sit every couple of minutes to bring her heart rate down. Dancing is extremely difficult, so we don't do much of that anymore.

We spend a lot of time going from doctor's appointment to doctor's appointment. Cardiology one day; pulmonology another day and oh wait, now to ENT and most recently to Neurology. Each time, the doctors are curious about her health issues, and still even after two years, they still continue to tell us that they just don't know how long all of these ailments will last or if they ever will go away. They continue to be stumped as to what to do next. It is all a mystery and an educated (or uneducated) guess as what to do moving forward.

One thing I do know, God has blessed us with more time together. I love her with all my heart, even more than I could have ever imagined thirty-seven years ago, and I will do anything that I need to in order to continue enjoying life together as we grow older. We have been blessed in so many ways.

It is funny from time to time, before she became sick, she would always say that I suffer from selective hearing, but now due to her occasional "brain fog," she is the one who does. Often, we will talk about something, and then five minutes later, she says, "Do you know what?" I tell her, "We just talked about that five minutes ago. Weren't you paying attention?" Well, I guess that is how I am being paid back after all these years.

This summer Lisa wanted to go back to CrossFit. We gave it three attempts. She didn't do too bad, but I told her she needed to start this out slowly. CrossFit at a regular interval, several times a week is a great goal for her to have, but for now, she is trying to find activities that she

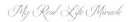

can do to strengthen her muscles and build endurance while allowing her not to achieve a high heart rate within one minute. CrossFit will come again someday, we hope.

We have only been shopping together twice in the past two years: to Target once and the grocery store once. Again, it is difficult for her to stand. Usually, she goes with me, but she waits in the truck with our dog, Harley, for me to shop and come back. It's not that she ever really enjoyed shopping; neither of us does, but we enjoyed doing it together.

Do I sit around moping about our ordeal with COVID? No! We both understand that it's God's plan and only He has control. There are some things which we have gained since Lisa became sick. First, our lives have finally slowed down a bit. We enjoy our coffee together in the morning a bit more. We enjoy the little important things like spending more time together reading or just doing nothing but being with each other, what they call "quality time." I have also started to realize that it's okay to ask for help, but most of all that you have to take time to enjoy life and enjoy those around you. Take time to enjoy the beauty of God's creations. Life is not just about "me."

We should be thankful for the time we have and be thankful for the people we have in our lives. We didn't know from day one what we would do for a living when we grew up or how we would spend the rest of our lives. God has the plan. But I do see now what He had in mind, and I am extremely thankful for that. My prayers are filled each day with thanks for allowing us to have more time together, with hope that Lisa's illness and our trials and tribulations will be a light for others who are experiencing illness and recovery to lean on God, and to cherish those important in your life. No one has to experience this alone.

God Really is in Control!

As I am writing this, the world seems to be imploding on itself. Inflation and gas prices are at an all-time high. Russia has invaded Ukraine. China seems like they are playing some sort of Hunger Games. Iran is on the hunt. North Korea is sitting back and watching how America responds. The Afghanistan withdrawal was a disaster. The current administration is weak, which is giving the rest of the world the opportunity to create havoc. We are heading toward a one-world currency. Let me mention those events again so you can see a clear picture:

COVID virus paralyzes the world;

Millions die from COVID;

Others suffer long term effects of COVID;

Uncle Joe wins the presidency;

Afghanistan withdraw was a disaster;

Russia invades Ukraine;

Inflation is the highest it has ever been;

Gas prices are higher than ever;

Supply chain issues leaving shelves bare—moms can't find formula for God's sake;

China and Russia are on the hunt;

Iran is on the hunt; and

North Korea is sitting by watching.

Many self-proclaimed prophets would say the end is near and that many of the signs of the end have come to pass as they were described in the book of Revelation. Perhaps that is so. But I do know one thing: God is in control. He is watching how we are making a mess of things here on the very earth He created in seven days. We have screwed it all up. We think we are in control of our destiny.

We think. We think. And then we think some more.

We really have no clue. God, our heavenly Father, is in total control and always has been. Do you remember what I talked about earlier when God had Noah build that ark? The forty-day flood that wiped everything out except what was saved inside the ark so He could start again? What makes you think we aren't heading toward something like that again?

When was the last time you heard him speak? When was the last time you sat quietly, just listening to Him? Have you *ever?* Would you know He was speaking to you? Do you have that child-like innocence like Samuel so you are in the perfect position to hear from him? If you haven't heard from Him in a while, perhaps it is time to start that intimate relationship with Him that He desires of us. Do you have even a mustard seed of faith?

Those little nudges you get are not *your* conscious. Nope, they are the Holy Spirit kicking you in the head, trying to get your attention. It's the Holy Spirit convicting you. Wake up! It's time, my friends, to sit quietly; and ask God to open your eyes, mind, ears, and hearts. Let Him in. He is really in control. God gives us everything we need to have a relationship with Him and to prepare ourselves to hear from Him, we just need to tap into it. We need to spend time reading the Bible, in prayer, and also sitting in the quiet so we can hear Him. It's there. I know you feel it.

Dust off those old Bibles and dive into His Word. If you don't know where to start, the beginning is always a good place to start. God has shown us in so many ways that He is still in control. That He wants to spend time with us. He wants us to seek Him out. Start your day by praying and end your day by praying. Having a conversation with the heavenly Father is the perfect way to start and end a hectic day. What better way to get yourself centered after a trying day than to spend time with the Father? He is waiting.

Worship Him. Thank Him. Pray those big, bold prayers. Then sit and pay attention. You may not see God at work right away, but you *will* start to recognize God at work in your life. It does not matter how you have lived your life up to this point; it just matters what you do next. God promises to provide to those that believe and have faith. Trust in Him. Have faith in Him. Believe in Him. He is waiting on you.

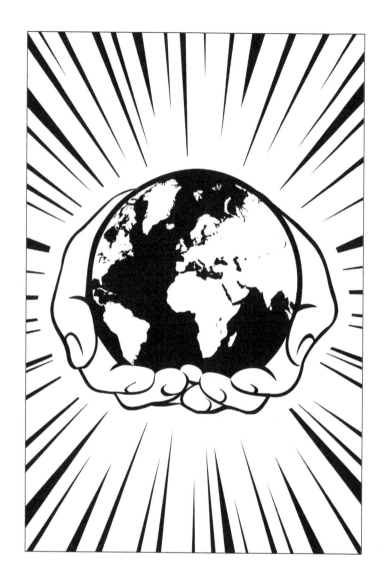

Where Am I Now?

Here I am, beginning year number three, and I am still a long hauler. I still suffer from POTs, shortness of breath, fatigue, hearing loss, and tinnitus. I still can't walk or stand for longer than five minutes. My regulator is still broken, folks. I am still working with reasonable accommodations. I only go in two days per week, but I honestly do not know how much longer they will allow me to do that. In fact, by the time you are reading this book, I might very well be retired on disability.

Every time I see the pulmonologist, he gives me another six months before he makes any decisions on my progress. He always tells us that I am in a difficult predicament. No one really knows what's next, what treatment modalities will work, and which ones will make things worse. There is really no cure that has been discovered. I often describe it as playing darts with a blindfold on. Just throw it and where it sticks is what we are trying this week. The cardiologist has already placed me at maximum medical improvement. He thinks since POTs has not resolved itself yet, it never will.

I took the first vacation in two years this past summer, and it was so hot that I could not really enjoy myself. It was great to visit with family, but it took me twice as long to recover from the fatigue. A second vacation to Key West with a small group of people was even more of a nightmare. There was nothing, and I mean nothing, that I could do that was easy on my body, as I am still a long hauler, still suffering from POTS, shortness of breath, weakness, and unable to stand or walk for longer than five minutes. My legs would scream at me, my heart would race, and my breathing was labored, all of which would cause me to sweat bullets. We rented a house on stilts, which meant so many stairs just to get in and out of the house. It took everything I had to climb and up and down those stairs. It felt as if I had exchanged one prison for another. Traveling to downtown where all the shopping and restaurants were located was a disaster. Parking was blocks away from the restaurants or shops we wanted to visit. Of course, that is the very thing I just can't do.

The shopping area was so crowded, and with our big, manly truck, we could not find parking anywhere close where the front or back end of the truck was not sticking out. It did no good for me to be dropped off in front of some place and wait while the truck was parked because standing is just as bad as walking. Hot, humid weather, sunshine, and Long COVID equals the perfect combination for my symptoms kick into full gear. Add in all the steps to the rental house, and it just helped create the perfect storm.

We had not seen the majority of these people who came on this trip since before 2020, so they had no idea what to expect when they saw me. I am sure my appearance was a shock. And, although they knew I was a long hauler, they had no idea how much of a toll these symptoms took on me nor how much they limited my activity on a daily basis. It is hard to explain to someone who has not lived this with us what it is like to live the life of a long hauler. When you turn on the news, you hear nothing but how the pandemic is over and we are now in the endemic phase; however, the pandemic is not over for us. We live it every day. Everyone else has moved on from the pandemic, grown into 2023, and here we are still stuck in 2020.

The world and our families have moved on, but we have not. Never in a million years could we have expected to be stuck in this, whatever this is, for this long, but here we are three years later. We are stuck and can't get out. There are few answers to our questions and no estimates on how long this will go on or how we even move forward from here.

We do the same thing day in and day out, not knowing how long we will continue this *Groundhog Day* experience. We don't make plans for the far-off future because there are too many unknown factors we would need to take into account, such as the weather, the environment, or even how I will be feeling at that time. It is just crazy to even try to explain it. Most of our family and friends have no idea what we have been going through. Most of our family or friends have not been around to witness the daily struggles that I have, and they could not even begin to guess what to expect when they see me for the first time.

After a day or two of not being able to do anything, I began to feel as if I had exchanged one prison for another. This one just happened to have a ton of stairs and beautiful, tropical weather. My heart rate and my breathing were out of control. We had a tiny bathroom that did not have good air flow, and the shower did not have a seat, causing me to stand the entire duration. This in turn, caused my heart rate to increase significantly. It took me hours to recover from just show-ering. Everyone else was ready to tackle the days adventures while I was just silently dying inside. I typically didn't start to feel anything close like my new normal self until the sun had gone down each day, and it started to cool off outside.

I know our group did not understand, and they just thought we were being unsociable, didn't want to do anything with them, or were just being plain difficult. We really weren't. The limitations and dis-abilities that I now have are very real, even though I may look perfectly normal on the outside. It isn't until you look close enough that you see the beads of sweat on my forehead or notice my erratic breathing and my gasping for breath. We used our dog as the excuse why we couldn't do what everyone else was doing because they just didn't understand. We made excuses why we couldn't do things so as not to bring atten-tion to my limitations and disabilities. I simply can't do that.

I had a healthcare provider recently tell me that COVID is in the past. It's time to focus on the present. She was my ENT provider. Notice I said "was." Yes, that's right; I won't be seeing her again. I have been seeing the ENT provider for my tinnitus and hearing loss. Compared to the other conditions I now have, that is the least of my concerns. I will admit that the tinnitus is driving me insane, but on the whole scope of things, it is the least important. People live with tinnitus for years, sometimes a lifetime, dealing with it.

We are taught in nursing school to focus on the ABCs first. That is airway, breathing, and circulation. Tinnitus is not impacting any of those functions of my life. And yes, I know, there have been some with tinnitus, who have committed suicide, so I do not take this condition lightly. Sometimes, I have a buzzing sound in one ear and a cricket sound in another. Some days it is so loud that I can barely concentrate or think straight. It keeps me up at night.

I have problems hearing a conversation when there are multiple conversations going on in a room at the same time. I often wonder if I am agreeing to something that is going to get me in trouble! A lot of times, I smile and nod, without having any idea what the other person is saying. I just let the cat out of the bag! Oops, sorry, folks; I'm just being real here. And it doesn't get any more real than this. I am a shadow of my former self.

That's right, a shadow of my former self, just a shell of the woman I once was. I look in the mirror and don't recognize the woman looking back at me. I see this stranger in the mirror who is frail, older-looking, and sickly. I see a train wreck. I know I have come a long way from where I was that dreadful night I walked into the hospital and even when I came home and for months afterward, but I still am not the person I once was. I can't do the things I once loved to do. I haven't been for a walk in the park in over two years. I have not walked my dogs in over two years. I haven't been for a walk around a campground with my husband in over two years. I have not done CrossFit in two years. I can't make my rounds at work like I used to in two years. I can't stand in church during worship and sing. I can't stand for longer than five minutes at a time.

I cringe every time someone stops me in the hall to chat. They may see the sweat beading up on my forehead and starting to drip down my face, which is so embarrassing, but they do not realize that I am dying inside. I have not cleaned my house in two years, though my husband has and continues to, as much as I hate that I can't clean my own house. Promise me you won't tell my husband. Ssshh—let that be our secret. I have not done much cooking in two years. I really miss that.

The positive side is that I am no longer on oxygen, and I can shower and dress myself without supervision. I just recently started driving myself to church, which is only about four miles from my house. I have not ventured any further than that alone. It is very difficult to press in my clutch. Actually, driving is just exhausting. I would rather not do it at all, to be honest. My husband has been driving Ms. Daisy around for over two years, and I am just as content right now to keep it that way until I can build the strength back in my quads and hamstrings. I yearn to have my full independence back, but I also don't want to do anything that is going to jeopardize my recovery.

I fully believe that I am going to continue to get stronger, but I am realistic enough to know that I won't be without limitations. Slow and steady wins the race, and I am in the race of my life. It's a marathon, not a sprint. No matter how much I want to force myself back to my former self, I know that is not possible. I must admit it is a hard pill to swallow. I would never admit this to anyone in my family, especially not my husband, so don't tell him, but I am probably one of the most stubborn, independent women ever! It's not in my nature to ask for help, to admit I can't do something or to depend on anyone else. In fact, I am known to do what you tell me I can't do. So, this is a new norm for me. It's out of my comfort zone, but I have not completely accepted this.

As a healthcare worker, I can understand that this virus has literally held the world hostage, not to mention the lives taken of so many people worldwide. It is new, and we just don't know enough about it.

But on the other hand, as a patient, this is truly frustrating. This has taught me that telling a patient, "We just don't know" is completely unacceptable. We deserve to be treated with dignity, respect, and we deserve, no, we demand to be believed. I am tired of being made to feel like a freak of nature by my own professional community.

I once had a Facebook friend tell me he thought COVID was made up by the government in an attempt to control us. I got angry and after cooling down a bit, my response was simply, "Come on, man! Seriously? Get real! Just take one good long look at me and what this has done to my life and tell me this is not real." Some people just can't help but be ignorant. What does he think—that this was a worldwide government conspiracy to control the entire world?

I don't know of one country that was not impacted by this virus. You will find COVID long haulers all over the world, not just in the good old US of A. But I know there are a lot of conspiracy theorists out there, who would rather believe that this virus is just a means created by the government to control us than to admit that God is real and that He really is in control. God could have stopped this virus from ever starting, but I think God needed to wake all of us up, myself included.

My nursing career is coming to an end, and I have come to grips with that. I know that must happen in order for me to continue to get stronger and to heal. I have learned so much about myself in the past two years and have grown so much. My faith has grown by leaps and bounds. While I feel COVID brain fog has made me dumb, I have also gained wisdom. I have learned not to sweat the small stuff. I have learned what is important in life. My relationship with my Lord and Savior and my family is what matters most.

My nursing career could care less if I am dead or alive. Your job will replace you in five minutes if you suddenly were not there. I have learned to put that into perspective. I no longer worry about things I have no control over. While I am sure I will miss the people I have come to know, I am sure I will not be missing the job. I know now to enjoy relaxing, traveling, and spending time with my family. I am now loving life. It's a life I would not have had without my own personal miracle. It saved my life.

It is extremely important to have faith and to believe beyond a shadow of a doubt that your dreams will come true. Everything is possible when you put your complete faith in God, when you open your heart and soul to have an intimate relationship with Him, and meet Him in that secret place, listening with an open mind, heart, and ears. Just invite Him into your heart and your life. Have you ever noticed those strange coincidences? Those are hints that He wants your attention. Listen. I promise it will be worth it. Miracles? Yes, those are real. They happen to everyday people all the time to people like you and me, everyday folks just trying to get by. Don't stop believing in yours.

Yes, the world has gone crazy. Yes, there seems to be more hate than love between people these days. Yes, we seem to have adopted a "instant gratification" mindset. I am just asking you to never stop believing. Yes, you might have hardships; God never promised the easy train, but He does promise everlasting life. He never told us we would not have sorrow or that life would be easy and that we will have everything we long for. If it is part of His plan for you, then it will happen in His perfect timing.

You might be led down a road with heartaches and disappointments; you might have financial struggles. You might experience health problems and struggles, but in all that, remember God has a reason for you to go through that. Have you ever heard that expression, "Pain lets you know you are alive?" I have always hated that expression, but it is very true. Thank God not only for your blessings but also your hardships. He has a plan and when the time is right, He will bring you into the Promised Land. He will bring you into all He has planned for you. Yes, He will. All you need is *faith*.

Don't stop believing. Just get to the place where you can easily say, "It is well with my soul" and mean it. Be the person that others can see God shine through you. Have a conversation with God every day. Praise Him daily. And don't be afraid to ask for favor, for strength, for health.

I know that I am not the only one this is happening to. There are several Long Covid support groups, different Facebook groups with millions of people around the world who are just like me, 17 million people to be exact. Just think about that number for a minute: 17 million people. That is the population of many entire countries. The fact that this virus paralyzed the entire world for well over a year and is still a factor in daily operations of businesses and countries should tell you something. This global pandemic impacted millions of lives. Oftentimes, we listen to the news about different tragedies happening around the world, and while we think how awful that must be, we truly do not grasp how awful it really would be to be impacted by a tragedy until it hits us personally. My family and I were no different. Now, our lives have drastically changed. We will not ever be the same people we were before 2020.

One thing this pandemic has taught us for sure is that we were not prepared. We are still not prepared. So-called Government's medical experts are biased to whatever political party's believe. They can be bought for a price. Fame and fortune are the two biggest roots of evil and control man. Medical experts, while they should be held to a different standard, are still human beings.

The lack of resources is still unreal almost three years later. Patients are still suffering; they still have no more answers than they had in the beginning. I have read so many stories from other long haulers and new symptoms they are experiencing with each passing day. It is heartbreaking that so many people are suffering. I just read about one woman who had a seizure at work and had to be transported to the emergency room. The seizure came from out of the blue, without warning.

I am not the only one; this is happening to millions of others across the world. I have been writing a blog, and several people have reached out to me to let me know that they have had similar experiences. I started the blog because you don't hear much about people like me. I knew the people suffering from long COVID had to be out there somewhere. Since starting my blog, I have joined a Facebook group for COVID Long Haulers, connecting others like me. I see new posts every day about a new symptom being experienced.

There are few research studies available at this point, making it hard for us to get answers. The lack of knowledge and resources for patients is making it difficult for us to get the necessary treatment. Long haul clinics are few, and those that are in existence are hard to get into. It takes months to get into one of these clinics and sometimes even longer. Physicians are reluctant to diagnose long haulers because of the lack of knowledge and resources available for them. How do we move forward from this? That is the million-dollar question.

The good news is I am not worse. I have been the same for quite some time now. So as long as I am not getting worse, I consider myself being "okay." The bad news is I am not getting any better. This just might be my new normal, and that thought really sucks. It sucks to think I won't do the things I love to do ever again.

God's Plan

As we have stated many, many times, our faith has been challenged throughout this entire ordeal. One would think, how in the world could this couple have faith and be thankful for what they have gone through? If we have learned anything at all through all of this, it is four significant things:

1. God is truly in control;

2. God has a plan for everyone;

3. You must have faith; and

4. It is never too late to start or renew a relationship with God.

I truly believe that all of this has not only strengthened our marriage and relationship, but receiving a renewed relationship with God has changed our lives forever. It has taught us to cherish each day, to slow down and enjoy life both physically and spiritually, cherish time with family and friends, and to cultivate a close relationship with God.

During the past two and a half years, we have spent countless hours traveling from doctors' appointment to doctor's appointment, this test and that test, and one specialist to another. Still there is much that the medical profession needs to learn about COVID-19, long haul COVID, and the treatment for both. This dreadful virus has completely changed everyone's lives. We have often described it as being held a prisoner of COVID. This past summer we went on a vacation with my sister and brother-in-law. We had this trip planned for quite some time. Lisa was very limited in what she could do. The heat and humidity of the South in August was unbearable for her. She very much wanted to sightsee and explore, but she was held back because of her many limitations and restrictions.

My sister and brother-in-law wanted to go-go-go but Lisa could not do that. It is hard for anyone that has not lived through this with us to understand exactly how this has impacted our lives and how she truly feels trapped inside this nightmare. She can't walk more than five to ten minutes without feeling dizzy, her heart racing, and before she starts sweating bullets. The way the weather affects her and restricts her even more is crazy. People on the outside of our little, tight circle just don't understand. We have tried to explain the impact this has had on our lives but it is hard for anyone to understand the changes to our lives COVID has had unless you have lived it with us. The only way to truly understand is to have known us prior to COVID, lived through this experience with us, and then perhaps you would understand how this has changed our lives.

It has had its devastating effects. Lisa can't do the things she loved to do. We can't do the things we loved to do. Something as simple as cooking together in the kitchen and perhaps dancing in the kitchen while cooking said dinner, is something we just can't do anymore. We both miss that terribly. We can't be spontaneous anymore. We just can't hop in the car for a road trip anytime we want. We just can't go to a concert or the beach. We can't sit outside in our own backyard in the summertime because it is too hot and humid for her to handle.

And though we have become frustrated from time to time due to a lack of answers as to whether her health will ever improve or is this our new normal life. Our renewed faith has seen us not only return to church, but she has become the Greeters Ministry Leader, responsible for greeting and establishing a welcoming presence to those new

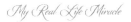

visitors as well as planning many social gatherings and potluck events. Lisa is also teaching one of the Women's Group Bible study classes each week. I facilitate the Senior Adult Bible study class. If anyone had asked me prior to her illness to teach a Bible study class, I would have told them to take a flying hike. But it didn't stop there. This past summer, I was asked to become an elder of our church. In July, I was ordained an elder and preached my very first sermon. What an *awesome* feeling that was and continues to be. We feel like our newfound faith has filled a void that our hearts have had for a long time.

She still has a long road ahead of her and we have unlimited questions regarding her chronic COVID Long Hauler illness such as "Will she ever get better?" "Will she get worse?" One thing that I do know for sure is that we are thankful for this second chance. Never squander the opportunities to praise God, love your family, and to take time marvel at all of God's creations. We pray every day for all the COVID long haulers that someday their questions will be answered, and cures will be found. In the meantime, we hope that each can find the peace and comfort we have found from our renewed faith.

God tells us that it only takes a mustard seed of faith. You can accomplish anything with only a mustard seed of faith. It doesn't require this massive amount of faith. Just a mustard seed sized faith. Our prayer is that this book gives someone hope for their future, that it gives comfort to someone in their time of need. Regardless of whether you struggle with a financial burden, health issues, unknown and difficult circumstances, or are just lost, we pray that our story helps you find the peace and joy you deserve through God's promise of love and eternal life. God loves you.

Lisa's Final Thoughts

This has been a very difficult journey for me and my family. I went from being healthy and active; my career full of promise and growth to being a shell of my former self. I must constantly monitor my heart rate and oxygen saturation. I am limited in my activity. Any kind of movement becomes exertion for my body and sends me into a tailspin. If the shuttle does not come to pick me up at work and I am forced to have to walk between my clinics, my legs scream at me, and it takes me days to recuperate. God forbid, I have to go in two days in a row. That is torture.

I was very strong before contracting COVID. Now my once muscular, strong legs are chicken legs. There is literally zero muscle definition in my legs now. Let's face it, my legs can barely hold my body upright. I can barely carry my own laptop or a grocery bag. Anytime I am horizontal, I sweat bullets which is absolutely the most embarrassing thing EVER. I am not a pretty sight when I am walking; sweating bullets, trying to breathe and waddling like a penguin. No, definitely nothing sexy about that walk. I was very independent prior to COVID and now I am anything but independent.

Yes, I am still working and thus far, I have been very fortunate to be allowed to work from home and only go into work two days per week but honestly even working from home is mentally and still physically exhausting. Oftentimes when I am talking, I can't remember what word I am looking for; can't remember the official terminology for things. It is so embarrassing to be as educated as I am and when in meetings, can't

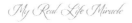

remember what things are called or what in the world I am talking about. I have shied away from any workgroups and from being called on by executive leadership because I am embarrassed, and I do not want to feel like a fool or be a disappointment. Just imagine being once highly sought after in your chosen career field, being considered a subject matter expert to suddenly praying no one notices you because you feel dumb.

The exhaustion I feel from little to no exertion takes such a toll on me; it is so very hard to describe. I have given birth to three children; two of which were cesarean births; I have participated in the CrossFit Open; I have done a 5K obstacle course and I have been a trauma nurse working twelve hour shifts and I have never in my life EVER felt this kind of exhaustion before. I fall asleep in the car on my way to work and on my way home. The post exertional malaise is unequivocally disabling.

When we were in Key West, I dreaded every time I had to go up and down those stupid stairs. Even going up and down out of the camper is difficult and exhausting. Walking from my office to the printer is exhausting; let alone getting to my office in the first place. My husband keeps threatening to take a video of me walking to my office so he can show it to the numerous physicians that I see how very hard it is on me.

My heart rate can go from 60 to 150 in a matter of minutes; then back down to 60 just as fast. It is scary. The sweat beads up on my forehead in a matter of minutes. My breathing becomes erratic in a matter of minutes. It does not matter if I am standing or walking. They are equally as bad. I dread every time someone stops me in the hallway to chat. I feel like I am dying inside. The best way to describe this is that I constantly feel like I am running a marathon. My heart races, my breathing become labored, I get dizzy, and I become utterly exhausted in minutes just by standing up.

My fight or flight is always triggered. I was once an adrenaline junky and now I can't handle the slightest amount of stress. It does not matter what it is or how minuscule it is, my body can't handle it. My heart rate races, my blood pressure soars, my head pounds; the chest pressure is unbelievable, and I feel physically ill. That takes me hours to recover from. There have been a few times when I was very upset or stressed that I almost felt it necessary to go to the emergency department- *almost.*

The symptoms of long COVID are debilitating and life changing. Living with long COVID is a challenge but one we will tackle. I am just so thankful He chose me. I know God has a purpose for my life and I am ever so grateful for that. That night, sitting in the dark in my room all alone with the machines beeping and my thoughts racing, I was comforted and for the first time, I knew God needed me for more. I had my Mary Magdalene moment that night. He sent me my angels to reassure me and to give me hope, and I was given the miracle of my life. I promised that night that I will honor God with my life, and I intend to keep that promise.

I have a scar on my left check from my ear to my jawline; my hair is coming in platinum grey, and I have a scar on my right buttocks from the skin breakdown that had started while in the hospital. These are my battle scars and I wear them proudly. Even my weak, chicken legs are a part of those battle scars and although I do get frustrated with them, I still try to stand up straight and am very honored to have been chosen to tell this story.

Thank you for taking this journey with us; for reading our story and we just pray that you find comfort in your own situation, no matter what it is from our journey. We implore you if you are struggling with your faith to find that tiny little mustard seed of faith, place your trust in God, dust off that old Bible and dig in. You won't regret it. Put on that armor of God every day and prepare to live your best life.

Thank you from the bottom of our hearts. God Bless each and every one of you.

Now Faith is confidence in what we hope for and assurance about what we do not see (Heb. 11:1)

CPSIA information can be obtained
at www.ICGtesting.com
Printed in the USA
LVHW072337090623
749373LV00008B/114